Phil Bonn
12/64

JOHAN L. SLOOFF, M.D.

SPECIAL APPOINTEE OF THE MAYO FOUNDATION, SECTION OF PATHOLOGIC ANATOMY, MAYO CLINIC, ROCHESTER, MINNESOTA, 1959–1961. PATHOLOGIST, KATHOLIEKE UNIVERSITEIT, NIJMEGEN, THE NETHERLANDS.

JAMES W. KERNOHAN, M.D., M.A.

EMERITUS CONSULTANT, SECTION OF PATHOLOGIC ANATOMY, MAYO CLINIC; EMERITUS PROFESSOR OF PATHOLOGY, MAYO FOUNDATION, GRADUATE SCHOOL, UNIVERSITY OF MINNESOTA, ROCHESTER, MINNESOTA.

COLLIN S. MacCARTY, M.D., M.S.

HEAD, SECTION OF NEUROLOGIC SURGERY, MAYO CLINIC; PROFESSOR OF NEUROLOGIC SURGERY, MAYO FOUNDATION, GRADUATE SCHOOL, UNIVERSITY OF MINNESOTA, ROCHESTER, MINNESOTA.

PRIMARY INTRAMEDULLARY TUMORS OF THE SPINAL CORD AND FILUM TERMINALE

W. B. Saunders Company / *Philadelphia* / *London* / *1964*

Primary Intramedullary Tumors of the Spinal Cord and Filum Terminale

PREFACE

FOR MANY YEARS our predecessors and associates have been interested in tumors of the spinal cord. During the last 30 years various studies of the clinical and roentgen-ray diagnosis, the surgical management, and the pathologic investigations of various types of tumors of the spinal cord have been reported. We wish to express our thanks to our predecessors, particularly W. D. Shelden, H. W. Woltman, A. W. Adson, W. McK. Craig, and J. D. Camp for their efforts in accumulating this abundant material and thus making this study possible. The present review is the culmination of the work of many members of the staff of the Mayo Clinic.

In the earlier years, when the basis for this study was laid, there were few aids to the diagnosis of tumors of the spinal cord, and detailed neurologic examinations were the only method of arriving at an accurate localization of such neoplasms. The surgical treatment was hampered by the difficulty of controlling bleeding and the ever-present danger of infection. These hazards are still present, but are greatly diminished, whereas accurate localization is now greatly aided by myelography. Bleeding is more readily controlled by electrocoagulation, and infections are held in check by chemotherapeutic and antibiotic agents.

We hope this report will be of service to all who have the care of patients with tumors of the spinal cord; the work is directed especially to neurologists and neurosurgeons, and to pathologists who report on the tissue removed. We also hope it will be of interest and help to all students interested in neurologic diseases.

We wish to express our gratitude to Mr. Louis W. Nichols, Jr., of the Section of Photography of the Mayo Clinic, for the preparation of all the photomicrographs; to the Section of Medical Illustrations for the preparation of the charts and tables; to the laboratory assistants in the Section of Pathologic Anatomy, and to Mrs. Beth Zimmermann for her secretarial assistance; and to Dr. James R. Eckman of the Section of Publications, for help, advice, and guidance in the preparation of the manuscript.

We finally express our thanks to the publishers for granting us the liberal use of illustrations. Without adequate illustrations, the usefulness of a volume of this type would be diminished. We are appreciative of their generosity in this respect.

JOHAN L. SLOOFF

JAMES W. KERNOHAN

COLLIN S. MACCARTY

ACKNOWLEDGMENT

One of the authors, J. L. Slooff, M.D., gratefully acknowledges a stipend received from the "Niels Stensen Stichting," Amsterdam, The Netherlands, which made possible his study at the Mayo Clinic, Rochester, Minnesota, from 1959 to 1961.

CONTENTS

I

Tumors of the Spinal Cord: General Aspects

INTRODUCTION

It can be assumed safely that the existence and clinical importance of tumors of the spinal cord have been known for several hundred years. It was not until 1887, however, that the first intradural but extramedullary tumor of the spinal cord was removed successfully by Victor Horsley, after the diagnosis had been established by Gowers.[106] It was another 20 years, in 1907, before the first intramedullary tumor was successfully operated upon by Eiselsberg [Eiselsberg-Ranzi[77] (1913)]. These two surgeons can be credited for the increasing interest in this previously hopeless condition. Their efforts proved that lesions of the spinal cord can be removed successfully without too much or even no damage at all to the function of the spinal cord.

The simplification and perfection of lumbar puncture by Quincke[220] in 1891 and the adaptation of lumbar puncture to the study of the hydrodynamics of the cerebrospinal fluid by Queckenstedt[219] in 1916, as well as the advance in roentgenologic technics and interpretation, have proved to be of considerable value in the establishment of an earlier and more nearly accurate diagnosis. These measures are welcome addenda to the clinician who is faced with the difficult problem of evaluating the significance of the various symptoms, such as pain, disorders of sensation, and disturbance of motor and sphincter function. The results of early surgical intervention are usually encouraging, since

1

intervention may bring about total restoration of function. For the ultimate prognosis, however, the surgeon often is dependent upon the histologic nature of the removed tissue. To the histopathologist, the microscopic examination often is appealing, since he is faced with tumors of many sources of origin, such as bony structures, cartilage, ligaments, fat tissue, lymphoid tissue, spinal nerve roots, blood vessels, meninges, cord tissue, and congenital rests. It is, however, at this point that the interest of clinician and pathologist often is divergent. The former is predominantly interested in the prognosis for his patient, and the latter, preoccupied with the great variation in cytologic and histologic structures of the tumors, is not easily satisfied.

As Bailey[13] (1938) pointed out, there are two possible bases for the classification of gliomas: (1) a practical viewpoint tending to result in a classification useful to the clinician; and (2) an academic viewpoint tending to result in a classification more meaningful to the biologist. In this study an attempt will be made to find some correlation between both viewpoints. For such a study, certain criteria and limitations must be set. Our purpose was to study primary intramedullary tumors of the spinal cord. It appears worth while to give some explanation of our understanding of this concept.

The commonly accepted grouping of tumors of the spinal canal is on the basis of location of the lesion in respect to the various structures which compose the spinal column. In this way one recognizes the intraspinal but extradural, the intradural but extramedullary, and the intramedullary locations. The intramedullary lesions can be defined as "lesions located in the substance of the medulla spinalis." The lesions of the filum terminale often are considered apart. Harmeier[118] (1933) divided the filum terminale into an intradural part and an extradural part. He wrote that the intradural part appeared to be composed of elements similar to those found in the other segments of the medulla spinalis, although there was a difference in the proportion of the constituent cells. Especially noted was the fact that there were less neural and glial tissue and relatively more ependymal cells. A similar predominance of ependymal cells also is noted in the conus medullaris, and this predominance appears to be the result chiefly of the presence of the ventriculus terminalis [Kernohan[140] (1924)]. There is no doubt that the conus medullaris is a part of the medulla spinalis. Why should we hesitate to accept the notion of the downward continuation of the conus medullaris, which is the intradural part of the filum terminale, as the lower extension of the medulla spinalis?

It seems logical, therefore, to include tumors of the intradural part of the filum terminale in a study of intramedullary tumors of the spinal cord.

In respect to the word "primary," we wish to qualify it by noting that we are dealing only with tumors which originated in the substance of the medulla spinalis and filum terminale. In most instances we had to base our opinion on the surgical reports or, in a small number of cases, on necropsy records. Those cases in which there was doubt regarding the original location of the tumor were not included in this study. It will also be understood that tumors originating from heterotopic glial tissue situated outside the medulla spinalis similarly were excluded.

The word "tumor" is used in the sense of "neoplasm."

INCIDENCE

Tumors of the spinal cord are considered to be rare. It is difficult to appraise accurately the frequency of occurrence of tumors of the spinal cord. When we began to evaluate the incidence, we found that this problem has been studied from different points of view by several authors.

One method of obtaining this information would be the study of a large group of postmortem examinations. This was done by Schlesinger[257] in 1898. He found 151 instances of intraspinal "tumors" in a series of 35,000 necropsies. Unfortunately, the word "tumor" at that time was used in relation to more disease entities—such as tuberculomas and gummas- than is true at present. In his series he found 20 intramedullary "tumors," but added that it was impossible to give exact figures concerning the frequency of occurrence of the gliomas, remarking, "There is no common opinion in regard to the meaning of the diagnosis glioma."

More information can be gathered from a study by Peers[212] (1936). In a series of 10,592 consecutive necropsies, 5150 examinations of the head were performed. There is no note as to whether the spinal cord was included routinely in the examinations. In these 5150 examinations 188 "tumors" of the central nervous system were encountered (this included 19 instances of tuberculosis and syphilis). There were 81 gliomas of the brain and four intramedullary neoplasms of the spinal cord (gliomas). Thus, we find that on this basis intramedullary tumors of the spinal cord represent 0.08 per cent of the total group of lesions found during examination (supposing that examination of the spinal cord was performed routinely), or 4.9 per cent of the 81 gliomas.

Flock[91] (1936–1937) found one glioblastoma of the spinal cord in 8172 postmortem examinations (0.01 per cent, or 1.3 per cent of 74 intracranial gliomas).

Courville,[55] according to Poser[217] (1956), found three intramedullary tumors in a series of 30,000 necropsies.

There is no doubt that a necropsy series, although it provides valuable information, cannot be regarded as completely representative of the incidence of any type of disease, since it is a well-known fact that the number of times permission for necropsy is granted is dependent chiefly on the special interests which certain conditions evoke.

A second way of obtaining some insight into the incidence of intramedullary tumors of the spinal cord is to compare the number of tumors of the brain with the number of tumors of the spinal cord seen by neurosurgeons.

Eiselsberg and Ranzi[77] (1913) described two intramedullary tumors of the spinal cord, as well as 183 tumors of the brain (this includes also nongliomatous tumors). Elvidge, Penfield, and Cone[84] (1937) found 20 gliomas of the spinal cord in a series of 210 gliomas of the central nervous system. Gagel[100] (1938), in a paper describing 237 gliomas of a group of 560 tumors of the central nervous system, mentioned that 11 gliomas were located in the medulla spinalis. Wolf (1941), in Elsberg's[80] *Surgical Diseases of the Spinal Cord, Membranes and Nerve Roots* (1941), reported the finding of 22 intramedullary gliomas as compared to 704 gliomas of the brain. These tumors were among 253 primary and secondary intraspinal neoplasms found at 4426 necropsies and among 2717 surgical specimens. Broager[31] (1953), in his study of neurilemmomas, reported that in a 17-year period 2548 intracranial (no further details were given) and 271 intraspinal tumors were found. Among the latter were 43 intramedullary gliomas (and 44 spinal neurilemmomas and 86 spinal meningiomas).

Table 1 indicates that there is a remarkable degree of difference between the frequency of occurrence of tumors of the brain and that of intramedullary tumors of the spinal cord. The figures of Eiselsberg-Ranzi[77] and of Broager[31] are comparable, since they deal with the total group of tumors of the brain. It is evident from these studies—and the view is acceptable—that there are one to two intramedullary tumors of the spinal cord for every 100 intracranial tumors. The difference in percentages in the series of Elvidge-Penfield-Cone[84] (9.5 per cent), of Gagel[100] (4.6 per cent), and of Wolf[304] (3.1 per cent) is remarkable and unexplained. No doubt it will be agreed that surgical series have a limited value, since they are influenced not only by the operability of the lesion, but by the interest of the surgeon in the particular lesion, and by his skill.

A third method of determining the incidence of intramedullary tumors of the spinal cord and one which, by reason of its objectives, is the most nearly ideal, deals with the frequency of occurrence of these lesions in a closed group of population. This was the objective of a study by Kurland[160] (1958). He used the resident population of Rochester, Minnesota, on the reasonable assumption that most people living there are attended during their illnesses by physicians of the Mayo Clinic. In a period of 10 years 50 intracranial neoplasms and 12 intraspinal tumors were recorded in a population of 30,000. During the calendar year 1954, 22 patients who had received the diagnosis of intracranial or intraspinal neoplasm were alive in this city. The number of these patients and age-adjusted rates pertaining to tumors in each site are shown in Table 2, which is taken from Kurland's paper.

The number of tumors of the spinal cord in the foregoing series is too small to be conclusive, so far as accurate determination of the incidence of intramedullary tumors of the spinal cord is concerned. Primary intraspinal neoplasms diagnosed in the 10-year period were classified as follows: three neurilemmomas, two meningiomas, and two ependymomas. One tumor was diagnosed on clinical and roentgenologic evidence only. There were four metastatic tumors inside the spinal cord. It thus can be expected that between 20 and 25 per cent of all primary spinal tumors are intramedullary in location.

Another and perhaps better approach to the relative incidence of intramedullary tumors of the spinal cord is study of published statistics from some of the larger series (Table 3). The available literature contains many, and some very interesting, incidental reports of cases, but they are not suitable as bases for evaluation of the frequency of occurrence of this type of tumor. Caution must be exercised in evaluating lesions in even the larger series, since the descriptions often are based on different criteria, with the result that, in some, metastatic gliomas and intramedullary vascular tumors are included with extramedullary vascular lesions. However, the difference between the two percentages for intramedullary tumors of the spinal cord shown in this table—10 in the series of Denk[68] and 23.4 in the series of Robineau[235]—is too extreme to be explained solely on this basis. We are unable to offer any explanation for this incongruence.

A few other facts can be found in Table 3. The generally recognized

Table 1. *Incidence, Based on the Literature, of Intramedullary Tumors of the Spinal Cord in Relation to That of Tumors of the Brain*

	Tumor, Site and Number		
Reporter	Brain	Intramedullary, Spinal Cord	Per Cent
Eiselsberg–Ranzi [77] (1913)	183	2	1
Broager [31] (1953)	2548	43 (gliomas)	1.6
Elvidge and associates [84] (1937)	210 (gliomas)	20 (gliomas)	9.5
Gagel [100] (1938)	237 (gliomas)	11 (gliomas)	4.6
Wolf [304] (1941)	704 (gliomas)	22 (gliomas)	3.1

Table 2. *Prevalence* of, and Age-Adjusted† Rates per 100,000 Population for, Neoplasms Affecting the Central Nervous System,
by Site, Population of Rochester, Minnesota, 1954,
Taken From Kurland*[160] *(1958)*

Neoplasm, Type	Patients, No.	Age-Adjusted Rate per 100,000 Population‡
Primary brain—certain	8	24.7 ⎫
Primary brain—probable	4	12.4 ⎬ = 46.0
Pituitary	3	8.9 ⎭
Intracranial metastasis	3	9.7
Primary spinal cord	4	12.9
All types	22	68.6

*Prevalence: the number of patients living at any time dur-
ing a specified year per unit of population; obtained by
accepting all patients who were resident and alive in
Rochester, Minnesota, at some time during 1954.

†Rate adjusted for age on the total population of the United
States in 1950.

‡Ninety-five per cent confidence limits of the age-adjusted
rates were computed.

Note: No patient for whom a diagnosis of intraspinal
metastasis had been made was alive during 1954.

predominance of males appears to be present in all the series represented
in which this information was given in the original paper. The ratio
which evolves from all the series in the table is that 14 males are affected
for every 10 females. A surprising observation arises when the several
rates of incidence are compared on the basis of the segmental location
of the tumors. Thus, the incidence of all tumors in the cervical segment
of the spinal column is seen to vary, among the different publications,
between 5.7 and 25.5 per cent, and the incidence of intramedullary
tumors in that segment is seen to vary between 17.3 and 75.0 per cent.
The same marked variation in incidence based on anatomic location is
noted in the thoracic (50.0 to 68.6 per cent for all tumors, against 19.1
to 80.0 per cent for intramedullary tumors) and lumbosacral (5.7 to 25.0
per cent for all tumors, against 1.4 to 51.7 per cent for intramedullary

Table 3.   *Relative Incidence, Based on the Literature, of Intramedullary Tumors of the Spinal Cord in Relation to all Spinal Tumors, With Indications of Sex of Patients and Location of Lesions*

Reporter	Total Spinal Tumors	Intramedullary		Sex		Cervical, Per Cent		Cervico-dorsal, Per Cent	Thoracic, Per Cent		Dorso-lumbar, Per Cent	Lumbosacral, Per Cent	
		No.	Per Cent	M	F	Total Group	Intramedullary		Total Group	Intramedullary		Total Group	Intramedullary
Denk[68](1932)	713	71	10.0	-	-	23.5	32.4	-	59.5	66.2	-	17.0	1.4
Eiselsberg[76](1931)	75	14	18.7	8	6	-	35.7	7.1	-	42.9	14.3	-	-
Jirasek[133](1932)	35	4	11.4	-	-	5.7	-	2.9	68.6	-	17.1	5.7	-
Robineau[235](1932)	64	15	23.4	8	7	15.6	20.0	-	62.5	80.0	3.2	18.7	-
Bunts[37](1935)	36	8	22.2	-	-	11.4	-	-	68.6	-	-	20.0	-
Foerster-Gagel[94](1935)	88	20	22.1	-	-	-	-	-	-	-	-	-	-
Ingebrigtsen-Leegaard[128](1939)	24	4	16.6	4	-	25.0	75.0	-	50.0	25.0	-	25.0	-
Elsberg[80](1941)	275	29	10.5	10	9	23.0	17.3	-	56.1	31.0	-	20.9	51.7
Woods-Pimenta[309](1944) lit.	-	-	-	72	54	-	29.0	9.5	-	51.5	2.5	-	7.5
Woods-Pimenta (1944)	-	-		18	17	-	25.7	11.4	-	28.6	11.4	-	22.9
Padberg-Davis[207](1952)	143	25	17.4	15	6	-	47.6	-	-	19.1	-	-	33.3
Henschen[121](1955) lit.	-	-	-	60	36	-	-	-	-	-	-	-	-
Henschen (1955)	-	-	-	-	-	-	34.3	-	-	47.4	-	-	18.3
Broager[31](1953)	271	43	16.0	-	-	18.3*	25.6	-	62.3*	34.9	-	19.4*	-
Ricard-Thiers-Bovet[228](1953)	206	26	12.5	-	-	25.5	-	-	56.0	-	-	18.5	-
Rogers[236](1955)	89	12	13.4	-	-	-	-	-	-	-	-	-	-

*Taken from 170 neurofibromas, meningiomas, and gliomas.

Table 4. *Incidence of Intramedullary Tumors of the Spinal Cord as*
Might Be Expected on the Basis of the Relative Length of the
Segments Compared With the Incidence of Lesions in
These Segments, Based on the Literature

Area	Expected Percentile Incidence of Lesions According to		Literature
	Root Level	Vertebral Level	
Cervical	23	22.5	17.3 to 47.6
Thoracic	58	51.5	19.1 to 80.0
Lumbar	19	26.0	1.4 to 51.7

tumors) segments of the spinal column. What is surprising is the observation that, although in the total group of spinal tumors the lesions
predominate in the thoracic segment (at least 50 per cent), this anatomic
predominance is not so pronounced in the case of intramedullary tumors
of the spinal cord. Surprising also is the high incidence of intramedullary tumors located in the cervical segment of the spinal column. It is
again emphasized that care must be used in applying these statistics,
especially since it is not certain whether or not tumors of the filum terminale are included in the several series.

According to Ravenel (cited by Elsberg[80]), the length of the cervical
portion of the spinal cord is 10 cm.; of the thoracic, 26 cm.; and of the
lumbar, 8.5 cm. On the basis of these data, 58 per cent of all tumors of
the spinal cord could be expected to arise in the thoracic, 23 per cent
in the cervical, and 19 per cent in the lumbar part of the cord. Approximately the same percentages (cervical, 22.5 per cent; thoracic, 51.5
per cent; and lumbar, 26 per cent) might be expected if the tumors were
to be situated on the basis of the vertebral level of the spinal column,
instead of the levels of the roots.

No definite opinions can be formed from comparison of these data
(Table 4), but it is open to speculation whether the incidence of intramedullary tumors of the cervical portion of the spinal cord actually is
relatively higher than would be expected.

Several studies have been made of intramedullary tumors among
children.

Review of the relative rates of incidence of gliomas in different studies
among children (Table 5) and a comparison of these with similar rates
among persons of all age groups (Table 3) might provoke speculation
whether the relative incidence of gliomas among children is slightly
higher than it is among adult persons, but the series are too small to
permit conclusions to be drawn in such a respect. According to some
authors [Hamby[116] (1944); Pasztor-Paraicz-Szénásy,[211] (1961)], gliomas are

Table 5. *Relative Incidence, Based on the Literature, of Intramedullary Tumors of the Spinal Cord Among Children*

Reporter	Total Group	Total Children	Intramedullary Gliomas	
			No.	Per Cent
Stookey [273] (1928)	165	8	3	37.5
Ingraham [129] (1938)	—	15	1	6.6
Hamby [116] (1944)	—	214	44	17.1
Buchanan [34] (1950)	—	6	2	33.3
Anderson-Carson [5] (1953)	—	22	9	40.9
Grant-Austin [108] (1956)	409	30	6	20.0
Ford [95] (1960)	—	23	5	21.7
Rand and Rand [222] (1960)	—	64	20	31.2

the lesions which occur most frequently among intraspinal tumors in childhood. This view, however, is not generally accepted [Ingraham-Matson[131] (1954); Krayenbuhl-Lüthy[158] (1947)].

ANALYSIS OF MATERIAL

In the appendix of this volume we are presenting the details of 301 cases of intramedullary tumors of the spinal cord, and in the text proper we present reports of 42 cases from among these 301 cases.

Slightly less than 10 per cent of all tumors seen at the Mayo Clinic are those which arise in the central nervous system and its coverings. Details are available concerning 8784 verified neoplasms in this category. About 85 per cent of these were located in the cranial cavity. They have been classified according to the histologic types shown in Table 6. Of this total group, 1322 tumors, or 15.1 per cent of all the central nervous system tumors, were located in the spinal canal. Histologically, these tumors have been separated into seven groups (Table 7). The largest group of these consists of neurilemmomas (383 cases, or 29.0 per cent),

Table 6. *Primary Tumors of the Central Nervous System Encountered at Mayo Clinic*

Gliomas	
Astrocytomas (grades 1 to 4)	2725
Ependymomas	283
Oligodendrogliomas	335
Medulloblastomas	184
Gliomas, type (?)	113
Neurilemmomas (intracranial)	617
Tumors of mesenchymal tissue	
Blood vessels	363
Sarcomas	241
Lipomas	7
Meningiomas	1493
Tumors of developmental defects	
Dermoid, epidermoid	94
Craniopharyngioma	196
Tumors of the pineal body	55
Tumors of the pituitary body	756
Tumors in the spinal canal	1322
(For specifications see Table 7)	
Total	8784

with a somewhat smaller number of meningiomas, and together they constitute more than half (721) of the 1322 intraspinal tumors.

The neurilemmomas were attached to the nerve roots, either intradurally or extradurally. Nearly two-thirds (62 per cent) were located intradurally, and this high percentage is partially explained by the fact that the dural attachment of the nerve root extends nearly to the dorsal root ganglion. Of the remaining, 6.2 per cent were both intradural and extradural, and 31.8 per cent were entirely extradural. Many of these latter were of a dumbbell shape, with the smaller portion within the spinal canal and the larger portion frequently being found in the thoracic cavity or, occasionally, in the retroperitoneal area or the abdominal cavity or, rarely, subcutaneously. The average age of the patients who had neurilemmomas was 43.5 years, the youngest being 11 months old and the oldest, 80 years old. The generally recognized preponderance of males afflicted with such lesions is also obtained in this series: there were 221 males and 162 females.

Characteristically, the neurilemmomas consist of interlacing bands of cells with elongated nuclei and parallel intracellular fibrils. The most specific finding is the tendency for the nuclei to be arranged in parallel rows—so-called palisading of the nuclei—and this type of tissue has been designated by Antoni as "type A." Unfortunately, many tumors may not have this characteristic appearance, and the picture may be mimicked by some meningiomas. Areas of loosely arranged tissue with many star-shaped cells simulating astrocytes may be present, and this tissue pattern has been designated by Antoni as "type B." Cells containing lipoid commonly are present, sometimes even in large numbers. Often small foci of degeneration and small cysts are found, and granules of hemosiderin occasionally are seen. The origin of neurilemmomas is still unsettled.

The 338 meningiomas in our series constituted 25.5 per cent of all the intraspinal tumors represented (Table 7). We found that 85.2 per cent of all the meningiomas were situated between the dura and the spinal cord. Slightly less than half of the remainder were both intradural and extradural, whereas the location of the other half was entirely extradural. The average age of the patients who had meningiomas was 49.9 years; the youngest patient was 3 years old and the oldest, 88 years. Meningiomas occur preponderantly among females; in our series 270 females were affected and only 68 males. Histologically, these tumors consisted primarily of groups of rather elongated plump cells with short

Table 7. *Histologic Classification of 1322 Tumors of the Spinal Canal, Mayo Clinic Series*

Type	No.	Per Cent
Neurilemmoma	383	29.0
Meningioma	338	25.5
Glioma (18 extramedullary)	291	22.0
"Sarcoma" (7 intramedullary)	157	11.9
Vascular tumor (10 intramedullary)	82	6.2
Chordoma	53	4.0
Epidermoid, etc. (10 intramedullary)	18	1.4
Total	1322	100.0

round or oval nuclei. The cells usually were shorter than those of the neurilemmomas, and, although interlacing bands of cells could be seen, there was a tendency toward the formation of concentric masses or whorls. Such a tumor is designated "meningothelious meningioma," and was the basic tumor of the group. Frequently in the center of the whorls calcification was present—the so-called psammoma body. Tumors with large numbers of these calcified bodies are designated "psammomatous meningiomas." In some cases the tumor consisted of predominantly fibrous tissue—the fibrous meningioma. Whether this fibrous tissue is the result of an overgrowth of the fibrous network of the meningioma, or is derived by neoplasia from the fibrous tissue of the arachnoid is difficult to determine. Very rarely are meningiomas developing in the spinal canal malignant.

The next group in order of frequency consisted of gliomas of the spinal cord (Table 7). There were 273 primary intramedullary gliomas, and they formed 22.0 per cent of all the intraspinal tumors in the series. Since they constitute the main subject of this study, the details referring to them will be described in the following chapters. Attention is drawn to the fact that 18 extramedullary gliomas (10 ependymomas and eight astrocytomas) were noted in our study. These tumors were separated from the larger group, because they originated outside the medulla spinalis, probably from heterotopic glial tissue. Some of these tumors were described by Cooper, Craig, and one of us (Kernohan[48]) in 1950.

The "sarcomas" listed in Table 7 were a mixture of different types of tumors: what they all had in common was origination from the intraspinal mesodermal tissue. In this group there were, for example, fibrosarcomas, lymphomas (those which had an origin in the intraspinal space), chondromas, and lipomas. Among these were seven with a primary intramedullary location—one sarcoma and six lipomas. There were 157 sarcomas of all types and various locations in the spinal canal, but only seven were inside the spinal cord. The 157 sarcomas of all types constituted 11.9 per cent of all intraspinal tumors.

The 82 vascular tumors, or 6.2 per cent of all the intraspinal tumors, consisted of tumors of blood vessels, both capillary and cavernous. The cavernous type of tumor rarely is removed at operation, so that histologic examples of this tumor are relatively few. Capillary tumors consisted of a few capillary hemangiomas with little evidence of neoplasia, and they were considered to be hamartomas. However, there was a much larger group of hemangio-endotheliomas and a smaller group of hemangioblastomas. Ten vascular tumors were limited to the substance of the spinal cord (Table 7). They will be described in Chapter III, "Vascular Tumors," p. 116.

There were 53 intraspinal chordomas (4.0 per cent). It would appear to be justified to include them as tumors of the spinal cord, since they develop from remnants of the notochord within the spinal vertebral column. The majority of them were found in the sacral region, but they were also present at other levels. Histologically these tumors consist of large spherical cells in a lobular arrangement, and they may be rather vascular. Characteristic is the "physaliphorous cell," a vacuolated cell which contains both glycogen and mucus. Usually, extracellular mucus also is present.

Nearly 1.4 per cent of all the intraspinal tumors were epidermoids, dermoids, or teratomas (18 cases) (Table 7). Ten of these were encountered in the substance of the spinal cord. The presence of these tumors may be explained on the basis of inclusion of ectodermal tissue during the process of closure of the spinal canal. The histologic picture of the intramedullary ones will be discussed in Chapter III, "Epidermoids, Dermoids, and Teratomas," p. 124.

In comparing the incidence of neurilemmomas, meningiomas, and gliomas on the basis of the vertebral level at which they were found, we noted that the percentage of the total count approaches fairly well the expected incidence (Table 8). The expected incidence on the basis of spinal segments for the thoracic level should be 51.5 per cent, and the actual incidence was 47.6 per cent. A complete comparison was hampered by the fact that the locations of some tumors crossed the borderlines between the several vertebral levels. A more nearly correct comparison could be approached by combining the tumors of the cervical, cervicothoracic, and thoracic levels (68.6 per cent) and comparing the incidence thus calculated with the expected incidence (74 per cent). The difference of 5.4 per cent does not seem to be significant. The same procedure can be followed in respect to tumors of the thoracic, thoracolumbar, and lumbar areas: the incidence in our series was 79.0 per cent, and the expected incidence was 77.5 per cent. The difference here—1.5 per cent—also does not appear to be significant. The fairly close agreement between the actual incidence and the expected incidence of tumors in a certain vertebral level seems to hold true throughout the total group, but attempts to find a similar correlation for the incidences of several individual tumor types are not similarly successful. As can be seen in Table 8, the frequency of occurrence of neurilemmomas in the thoracic area is about equal to that in the lumbar area, whereas the incidence would be expected to be higher in the thoracic area. A readily available explanation is that the length of the posterior nerve roots in the lumbar area exceeds significantly that of the thoracic nerve roots. There is no explanation at the moment why meningiomas should preponderate in the thoracic segment (81 per cent). Similarly, the reason for the higher incidence of gliomas in the lumbar area remains obscure.

Henschen[121] (1955) speculated whether the tendency of neoplasms (Gliombereitschaft) to develop in the medulla spinalis was less than the tendency for them to develop in the brain substance, even when consideration is given to the difference in the weight of these structures.

Table 8. *Incidence of Neurilemmomas, Meningiomas, and Gliomas on the Basis of Vertebral Level at Which They Occurred*

Lesion	Vertebral Level									
	Cervical		Cervicothoracic		Thoracic		Thoracolumbar		Lumbar	
	No.	Per Cent	No.	Per Cent	No.	Per Cent	No.	Per Cent	No.	Per Cent
Neurilemmoma	88	23.3	3	0.7	125	33.4	9	2.3	152	40.3
Meningioma	43	13.4	10	3.1	261	81.0	2	0.6	6	1.9
Glioma	34	13.9	20	8.2	63	25.7	63	25.7	65	26.5
Total	165	17.5	33	3.5	449	47.6	74	7.8	223	23.6

To confirm this supposition we measured the weight of the brain in patients between 18 and 65 years of age in whom no gross abnormality of the brain was known. In the same cases we also measured the weight of the spinal cord. The average weight of the brain in 100 consecutive cases was 1401 gm., and the average weight of the spinal cord was 37 gm. It thus appears that the weight of the spinal cord amounts to 2.57 per cent of the total weight of the central nervous system. In our series of primary tumors of the central nervous system there were 3640 gliomas of the brain substance and 273 gliomas of the medulla spinalis. Gliomas of the spinal cord also constitute 7 per cent of the total number of gliomas of the central nervous system; the expectation would be 2.57 per cent. In an effort to explain this percentage, which is almost three times higher than would be expected, it becomes apparent that ependymomas occur relatively more frequently in the medulla spinalis than in the brain substance. One hundred sixty-nine of a total of 452 ependymomas of the central nervous system, or 37.4 per cent, were found in the spinal cord and filum terminale. Even if ependymomas of the filum terminale (99 cases) are subtracted, the incidence of these ependymal tumors in the spinal cord (15.5 per cent) is still higher than would be expected on the basis of comparison according to weight.

In our series there were 2725 astrocytomas of the brain substance and 86 of the medulla spinalis, including the filum terminale; converted to percentages, astrocytomas of the spinal cord formed 3.05 per cent of all astrocytomas of the central nervous system. This percentage appears to be in close agreement to that which would be expected on the basis of comparison of weights (2.57 per cent) of these tissues. The percentage of oligodendrogliomas located in the spinal cord (eight cases, or 2.3 per cent of the total group of oligodendrogliomas of the central nervous system) appears to be in fair agreement with the 2.57 per cent that would be expected. The number of oligodendrogliomas situated in the spinal cord (eight cases), however, is too small to make the percentage significant. Our conclusion is that the tendency for ependymomas to develop in the spinal cord is remarkably greater than the tendency for them to develop in the brain substance. The tendency of astrocytomas and oligodendrogliomas to develop in the spinal cord is about equal to the tendency for them to develop in the brain.

SYMPTOMATOLOGIC FACTORS

It is not our intention to give a detailed description of the symptoms and signs of tumors of the spinal cord, but it does appear worth while to summarize leading aspects of the clinical picture. A detailed analysis of our cases, as well as representative reports of cases, will be included in the description of several tumor forms.

Nonne[202] (1913) expressed the opinion that there is no sign pathognomonic of an intramedullary tumor of the spinal cord. Nevertheless, the common opinion at this time is that a complete examination is likely to offer a fairly accurate diagnosis or a good probability that such a diagnosis can be established.

The symptoms and signs can be divided and will be described herein under the following headings: (1) history, (2) clinical findings, and (3) laboratory investigations.

History

Study of the literature brings out the fact that, although there is no general agreement on the point, pain often is the first and most prominent sign of a tumor of the spinal cord. In the series of Foerster and Bailey[93] (1936) the patients in 55 of the 100 cases studied reported pain as the first symptom, and Austin[6] (1960) found that 64 per cent of patients with intramedullary tumors in his series experienced pain as a major symptom. In our own series we found that 68.1 per cent of the patients with intramedullary tumors reported pain as the first sign of their disease.

The pain associated with tumors of the spinal cord is regarded chiefly as being caused by involvement of or traction upon the dorsal nerve roots, and, as the size of the tumor increases, pain also can be the result of pressure upon or irritation of the anterolateral tract of the spinal cord. However, the foregoing does not appear to be true in all cases of intramedullary tumors, and, as Austin points out, the mechanism of the pain in these cases often is obscure. He suggested as a possibility involvement of or pressure upon the nerves of the pia. In a clinical experiment involving stimulation of the spinal cord under surgical conditions of local anesthesia, he showed that pain always can be produced by stimulation of the dorsal roots, frequently by stimulation of the dorsal column, and rarely by stimulation of the spinothalamic tract. Sometimes, also, stimulation of ventral roots is effective in producing pain. Austin also mentioned additional mechanisms, such as facilitation and a decrease in inhibition or efferent discharge, as possible explanations of pain in diseases of the spinal cord.

The character of the pain appears to be variable, and many descriptions are found in reported cases, such as continuous or intermittent pain, lancinating pain, dull pain, and so on. Hence, it cannot be said that there is a specific type of pain.

Location of the pain can provide valuable information about the level at which the tumor involves the spinal cord. This is especially true if the pain is of the so-called nerve-root type and has the specific distribution of a particular nerve root or combination of roots. Thus, tumors of the cervical region of the spinal cord can cause pain that is localized in the neck or extends into the occiput, shoulders, or upper extremities, depending upon the exact location of the tumor. Lesions of the thoracic segment of the spinal cord can produce pain which frequently simulates intercostal neuralgia and the pain of cholecystitis, cholelithiasis, renal colic, and so on. This seems to be the reason why a significant number of patients who have tumors of the spinal cord undergo abdominal operations before the real origin of their pain is found. Tumors in the lumbar area often give rise to pain which resembles that of sciatica, and confusion of the pain caused by intraspinal tumors with the pain caused by herniated intervertebral disk is fairly common.

Often, however, the pain manifests itself as a vague, but fairly persistent, pain in the back, and in such an event it is much more difficult to interpret than it otherwise would be. It is also not uncommon for the pain of intraspinal tumors to commence in some region of the back and to spread later in the disease process to a specific peripheral region. On the other hand, the converse also is often encountered, meaning that the pain originates somewhere in the periphery and later becomes localized in the back. Sometimes the pain is not even persistent, but is intermittent, with long intervals in which the patient is free from pain and which can precede the other symptoms of involvement of the spinal cord for a long time.

Although pain certainly is highly subjective, several characteristic features of it often can be demonstrated. That is, a characteristic of the spinal pain which is peculiar and typical is that it is aggravated by coughing, sneezing, lifting, and straining at stool. This type of pain also often awakens the patient some hours after he has gone to bed. A plausible explanation for these effects was given by Eaton[72] (1941). The epidural space, between the dura on one side and the bone and ligaments on the other side, is composed of loose connective tissue and blood vessels. The veins of this area are directly continuous, by way of the intervertebral veins, with the retroperitoneal and retropleural veins. If the intra-abdominal pressure or the intrathoracic pressure or both is increased sufficiently, as in the case of coughing, sneezing, lifting, or straining, the veins surrounding these cavities will be compressed, and the outflow of the epidural veins, via the intervertebral veins, will be obstructed or slowed. This results in temporary venous congestion which displaces the dura toward the spinal cord and exerts traction on the nerve roots. The nerve roots may even be compressed by the surrounding veins. It is thought that this traction on or compression of the nerve roots produces pain only when the nerve root is affected by a disease process. Even in an instance of intramedullary tumor it is acceptable and understandable that replacement of or abnormal traction on the nerve roots is sufficient to cause a sensation of pain.

Eaton also offered an explanation for the pain which is experienced at night. He showed with roentgenologic measurements that the spinal column tends to shorten during daytime, as a result of compression of the intervertebral disks by the weight of the body. In a horizontal position the spinal column gradually lengthens again. This consequently changes the relationship of the spinal cord and its roots to the bony structures, and stretches the nerve roots slightly, causing pain if the roots are, or the spinal cord is, diseased. This pain can be so severe that patients often are forced to sleep in an upright or sitting position.

A really confusing factor sometimes found in the history is that this pain is precipitated by recent trauma or is related to remote trauma. Sometimes the pain has subsided for some time and has returned later. Some authors use this experience as a basis for the conviction that trauma is in some way a factor in causation of the tumor. It would appear, however, to be more logical to assume that the trauma precipitates the symptoms by causing something like, for example, a readjustment of the pressure of the cerebrospinal fluid or edema or hemorrhage in or around a previously asymptomatic tumor. In a remarkable number of cases signs of an old hemorrhage are found histologically, and it is conceivable that regression of these more acute changes is responsible for the temporary regression of the symptoms, causing the symptoms to become more intermittent.

Similar types of intermittent symptoms characterize the rare condition which is described as "spinal subarachnoid hemorrhage." Wyburn-Mason[310] (1944) described this condition in cases of arteriovenous aneurysm or of abnormal spinal arteries. Fincher[89] (1951) observed the same syndrome, although in a less severe and less violent degree, in five cases of intramedullary tumors of the lower part of the spinal column. The main symptoms of severe headache, meningeal irritation, sciatica, or paralysis or sensory disturbance in some part of the body below the head associated with bloody cerebrospinal fluid, may be the results of the occurrence of hemorrhage in the subarachnoid space. Since, when vascular disturbance is present, the origin of the bleeding is arterial, the fatality rate accompanying this condition can be better appreciated. When tumors of the spinal cord are present, the bleeding is thought to be venous in origin, the symptoms are less severe, and the attacks occur repeatedly without being fatal. The hemorrhage is thought to originate from the congested pial vessels, which rupture easily, especially under the stress of violent physical effort.

The preoperative duration of the symptoms is very variable, as will be seen in the next chapters. The nonspecificity, the intermittent occurrence, and the vague character of the symptoms are in large part responsible for this. The variable duration of symptoms also is caused by the slow progression of the signs, a rate which depends largely on the slow growth of the tumor itself. The rate of growth of the more malignant tumors is considerably higher, and the progression of symptoms consequently is much faster. Theoretically, the location of the tumor also can be held to be responsible for the preoperative duration of the signs, since the inner diameter of the thoracic portion of the spinal canal is known to be the smallest, and it thus permits less expansion of the spinal cord than in other sectors.

In slightly less than 30 per cent of the cases the first symptom of a tumor of the spinal cord is related to a motor or sensory disturbance. In 16.6 per cent a disturbance of motor function appears first, and in 10.6 per cent some kind of sensory disturbance is the first sign of the disease. In only 2.6 per cent of cases is dysfunction of the bladder or bowel the initial symptom. Since these are also objective symptoms, they will be dealt with more extensively in the next paragraph.

Clinical Findings

In a great number of cases the pain has not been recognized by the patient or his physician as the sign of a tumor of the spinal cord. The development of motor or sensory dysfunction or dysfunction of the bladder and bowel directs the attention to a more serious illness. It is impossible to evaluate what the next most important sign is, since in most cases what the physical examination brings out is chiefly a mixture of disturbances, some of which have escaped the attention of the patient. This usual course is understandable, for in nearly 70 per cent of the patients the development of these signs is the expression of progression of the tumor. The symptoms are totally dependent on the location of the tumor in the substance of the cord. It is, however, not only the physical presence of the tumor which produces the symptoms, but rather often accompanying changes, such as edema, vascular disturbances, and hemorrhages, which are thought to be at least partially responsible for the symptoms of the progression.

The character of motor involvement is described differently by patients, who may report weakness, clumsiness, stiffness, limp, and so on. Clinically, the motor findings can be divided into two groups: those which result from disturbance of the corticospinal tracts, and those which are the result of damage to the motor neurons themselves. In the first group the characteristic symptoms or signs are spasticity, spastic paralysis, exaggeration of the tendon reflexes, clonus, presence of the Babinski reflex, and the absence of muscular atrophy. In the second group the signs are hypotony, flaccid paralysis, loss of tendon reflexes, and signs of atrophy of the muscles supplied by the destroyed neurons. This latter group of signs usually gives a fair indication of the level of the lesion, whereas in the former group the signs are less specific in indication of the site of the tumor. Difficulty of interpretation also arises when the symptoms are in an early phase of development. As can be understood, the involvement need not be extensive, and in many cases only an occasional muscle or muscle group may be affected.

Additional help sometimes can be found in disturbance of the sensory functions, when such is present. Disturbance of this function frequently is described as numbness, tingling, cold feeling, hypesthesia, or complete anesthesia in a specific area. The type, extent, and location of the disturbance again are determined by the site and size of the tumor. Lesions in the central gray matter involving the commissure cause analgesia and thermanesthesia on both sides of the body, since they interrupt the spinothalamic fibers as they cross the midline. Lesions located in or extending into the posterior gray matter or at the site of entry of a nerve root cause anesthesia of segmental distribution. If the lesion is entirely confined to the gray matter, a condition which seems to be rare, there may be analgesia and thermanesthesia without loss of the tactile function. Lesions located in the posterior columns of the spinal cord give rise to ataxia, loss of sense of passive movements, loss of position, vibratory and two-point sense, and stereognosis on the ipsilateral side. Involvement of the zone of entry of a nerve root also may cause loss of tendon reflexes. It is the upper level of sensory disturbance which most often gives valuable information about the location of a tumor, but unfortunately this level is not always clearly demarcated. An important sign which directs attention to a lesion of the spinal cord is the inequality of the symptoms on both sides of the body.

Interference with the sphincters of the bladder and bowel was present as the first symptom in about 3 per cent of our cases, and in many more patients we find this symptom developing fairly early in the disease process. Unfortunately, it does not give information about the location of the lesion, but according to many authors, when this type of interference appears very early, it is indicative of a distal location of the tumor.

Richardson[229] (1960) pointed recently to the importance of spinal rigidity, usually associated with irritability, in the formation of an early diagnosis, especially in children.

The presence of kyphosis, scoliosis, or the combination of both is of little help in the diagnosis, although these conditions can be the results of the disturbed function of the spinal cord.

A very confusing symptom occasionally found in patients who have tumors of the spinal cord is the bilateral papilledema. We found nine examples in this series of intramedullary tumors. Three patients had an astrocytoma in the cervical portion of the cord; three patients had an ependymoma in the thoracolumbar and lumbar segments of the cord; one patient had an oligodendroglioma in the lower thoracic portion of the cord and another patient had a spongioblastoma in the cervical part of the cord. In one patient who had been operated upon for an oligodendroglioma in the mid-dorsal area, marked papilledema developed before death, whereas at necropsy involvement of the brain was not found. Papilledema is observed in the presence of tumors of the cervical area, as well as tumors of the thoracic or lumbar portions of the spinal cord. It disappears rapidly after surgical removal of the tumor. The mechanism of development of choked disks is not known, but the general impression conveyed in the papers available is that it is an evidence of increased intracranial pressure. This is in agreement with the often-accompanying internal hydrocephalus sometimes observed. There is considerable doubt about the origin of the increased intracranial pressure in tumors of the spinal cord, and several theories exist. Factors mentioned in several studies are disturbance of circulation of the cerebrospinal fluid, disturbed equilibrium between the production and resorption of cerebrospinal fluid, and increased protein content of the cerebrospinal fluid causing either elevated osmotic activity or partial obstruction of the absorptive areas of the cerebrospinal fluid which results in an increase in volume and pressure. It is doubtful, however, whether any of these causes constitutes the only one, since there are many more tumors of the spinal cord which cause obstruction to the circulation of the cerebrospinal fluid or which are accompanied by an extremely high protein content of the cerebrospinal fluid without producing any sign of papilledema. In our nine cases we were unable to find an additional factor which would offer a reasonable explanation.

Laboratory Findings

A necessary procedure, when the suspicion of a tumor of the spinal cord has arisen, is the performance of lumbar puncture. The data provided by this procedure can be very helpful in the decision as to the final diagnosis, and often are the bases for performance of laminectomy.

The first possibility, after the needle has been placed in position, is a so-called dry tap, meaning the inability to obtain cerebrospinal fluid. This phenomenon is encountered only if the tumor completely fills the subdural space at the level of puncture, and it results from the absence of fluid at this level. Repeated puncture at a higher interspace often produces the desired result unless the tumor is very extensive. Measurement of the initial pressure of the cerebrospinal fluid is the next step. In some cases the pressure is found to be extremely low, and it does not react to fluid-raising maneuvers, such as compression of the jugular veins. In these circumstances an obstruction can be expected to be situated above the level of puncture. Collection of the fluid yields only a small amount. The initial pressure also may be at a reasonable level, but may not react to jugular compression. In this situation the obstructing lesion more probably is situated at some distance from the level of the puncture. Another possibility, after the finding of a reasonable initial pressure, is a slow increase after the Queckenstedt[219] procedure or a normal increase but a slow decrease after release of compression of the jugular veins. All these events indicate a partial or near-total obstruction to the circulation of the cerebrospinal fluid.

Examination of the cerebrospinal fluid itself is of considerable value.

The findings commonly encountered are known under the names of several syndromes: "dissociation albumino-cytologique," which indicates an elevated protein content of the cerebrospinal fluid without an increase of the cells. The Froin syndrome indicates essentially the same, but adds xanthochromia. Elevation of the protein content is a very significant finding. Complete data were available in 146 cases in our series. The average value for protein content was 935 mg. per 100 cc.; the highest value for protein which we found in this series was 10,000 mg. per 100 cc., and the lowest was 10 mg. per 100 cc. The average cell count in these same cases was 6 cells per cubic millimeter of fluid. Complete block of the circulation of the cerebrospinal fluid was noted in 76 patients, and in 27 incomplete block was found. Detailed figures concerning these data will be found in the clinical reviews.

SURGICAL TREATMENT

Pathophysiologic Aspects

The neurosurgeon must have a basic understanding of the pathologic aspects of intramedullary tumors of the spinal cord if he is to manage these neoplasms intelligently by surgical means. He must understand the mechanisms which produce dysfunction of the spinal cord. Essentially it would appear that two fundamental processes cause disruption of the function of the spinal cord. They are: (1) simple compression of the cord exerted by the mass of the neoplasm, or coincidental compression of the adjacent blood supply with resultant destruction of the neurogenic elements of the spinal cord, and (2) actual replacement of the spinal cord by neoplastic tissue, with resultant interruption of nerve transmission. The first type of phenomenon is most likely to occur when an intramedullary lipoma, epidermoid, dermoid, or teratoma is present, as well as in the presence of many instances of ependymal-cell tumors. The second phenomenon is most likely to occur when neoplasms of the astrocytic series are encountered. Both phenomena may accompany all types of intramedullary neoplasms as the bulk of the tumor enlarges.

Location

The location of an intramedullary tumor is perhaps the most decisive factor in surgical therapy. The chances of successful and complete removal of an ependymoma of the cervical cord are remote. However, many ependymomas of the filum terminale can be completely excised without producing neurologic deficits. Thus it is apparent that tumors of the spinal cord in the cervical area are associated with risk, particularly in the matter of mortality. Tumors situated below the cervical area present a decreasing risk to the patient's life, but even so, neurologic complications persist as a hazard, particularly when these tumors are encountered in the thoracic and lumbar areas. The mortality and morbidity rates associated with the surgical treatment of tumors of the filum terminale are appreciably lower.

Types

Primary astrocytomas of the spinal cord are treated by wide and long laminectomy in an endeavor to overcome obstruction of the subarachnoid space by the swollen, tumor-bearing portion of the spinal cord. Postoperative irradiation therapy seems to be beneficial in many instances. Intramedullary ependymomas present a somewhat different problem. Longitudinal myelotomy between the posterior columns can be accomplished, so that part of the neoplasm arising from the central area of the canal can be exposed. The bulk of these neoplasms frequently can be removed. Postoperative irradiation therapy also seems to be beneficial.

In the experience of one of us (MacCarty[188]) tumors arising from inclusion cells, such as dermoids and epidermoids of the spinal cord, sometimes can be evacuated, but in many instances portions of the capsule which are intimately attached to the cord must be left behind. Because these neoplasms most often develop in the conus or cauda equina, the risk to life involved in removal of such tumors is not great, but neurologic defects usually are present prior to the operation and may be aggravated by excision of these relatively benign lesions. Dermoid tumors, in particular, may be associated with a dermal sinus, and are more frequently diagnosed during the victim's childhood or adolescence. Epidermoid tumors are rarely associated with dermal sinus, and therefore as a rule are diagnosed later in the patient's life. Another factor may be the characteristic slower growth of the epidermoid tumor.

Lipomas [Ehni[74] (1943)] which arise subpially present a special problem unless the site of origin and pathologic nature of the lesions are fully known and appreciated. Because they are intramedullary, meaning that strands of the tumor extend into the substance of the cord, they cannot be completely excised without destruction of tissue of the spinal cord. However, occasionally the bulk of the neoplasm can be reduced by removal of the superficial aspects. Wide and long laminectomy is desirable to overcome secondary compression of the cord and the blood supply of that structure. Postoperative irradiation is of doubtful value.

When a tumor of the filum terminale is at hand, the problem is less complicated because the tumor thus presents itself more or less as an extramedullary tumor. Consequently, if the neoplasm is recognized before severe neurologic disability occurs, the chances of a gratifying result are appreciably improved. As indicated previously, ependymomas are the intramedullary tumors most frequently encountered in this area.

Definitive Surgical Procedures

Diagnostic Methods (Surgical).   Roentgenologic examinations of the spinal column may be sufficient to locate an intraspinal neoplasm if the tumor has become sufficiently large to erode the spinal canal. Often, erosion of the facets, neural arches, and vertebral bodies may be seen in plain roentgenograms of the spinal column. In many instances, however, the tumor may be manifest clinically without producing discernible changes in the ordinary roentgenogram of the spinal column. In these instances it may become necessary to outline the neoplasm by myelography. It is imperative for the surgeon to know the location of the neoplasm and if possible to ascertain the longitudinal extent of it. If complete subarachnoid obstruction is present, the upward extent of the tumor may not be defined. Under these circumstances the surgeon must be prepared to perform long laminectomy. This is particularly true when the lesions are ependymomas, which may extend over the entire length of the spinal cord from the medulla to the conus.

Generally, myelography is performed through the lumbar subarachnoid space. Cisternal myelography can be done if it is necessary and desirable to obtain knowledge of the upward extent of the neoplasm in instances of complete subarachnoid obstruction. Occasionally the extent of tumors of the filum terminale can be determined by the simple expedient of performance of differential spinal punctures. If a complete block is present, as indicated by the Queckenstedt test when the needle is inserted at the fifth lumbar interspace, needles can be introduced into the canal at graduated upper levels until the block no longer is present, and in this manner the approximate extent of the neoplasm can be determined. While the diagnostic importance of contrast myelography is acknowledged, it is nevertheless true that the technic must be used judiciously. It can be dangerous [Hurteau and associates[127] (1954)]. There is accumulating evidence that radiopaque oil, when introduced into the subarachnoid space, may in rare instances cause death from acute aseptic purulent meningitis, or a less dramatic but definite chronic adhesive type of arachnoiditis. Thus we use myelography when other methods, both clinical and radiographic, are not of sufficient diagnostic accuracy.

Most intramedullary tumors do not contain calcium in sufficient amounts to be detectable at roentgenologic examination. Radiolucent areas reputedly are seen when the fat content of tumors is high. As a rule, however, neither the lipomas nor the teratomatous tumors can be detected by simple radiography.

Decompression.   Intramedullary tumors of the astrocytic type which occur above the filum terminale cannot always be completely removed without irreparable damage to the involved portion of spinal cord. As a consequence, about all that can be accomplished in many instances is biopsy and wide decompression. Sometimes even biopsy is too hazardous, as when the tumor is in the center of the cord. In that event damage would be done to functioning elements of the cord by attempts to reach the neoplasm. It is ordinarily safe, however, to insert a small needle into a swollen cord to identify a cyst or syringomyelitic cavity. Adequate decompression must overcome the obstruction to the canal, allowing for postoperative swelling of the cord and any residual portion of the neoplasm. This entails laminectomy carried out well above and below the tumor. It likewise means that the dura must be left open. If so, bleeding can be controlled more easily if the dural edges are sutured to the tissues near the edges of the laminectomy. It may or may not be desirable to cover the cord with a dural patch. In recent years we have used a homologous dural graft for this purpose. Hemostasis must be accurate to prevent postoperative hemorrhage and subsequent compression of the cord. Drainage of such a wound is con-traindicated because it might initiate a cerebrospinal-fluid fistula.

Subtotal Removal of Gliomas.   Occasionally an astrocytoma will appear on the surface of the cord and will appear to be almost encapsu-lated. It never is. However, the external portion of the tumor frequently can be excised under these circumstances without injury to the cord. Sometimes such tumors presenting on or near the posterior columns can be approached by longitudinal myelotomy, and a large portion of the gliomatous tissue can be removed, thus decompressing the cord.

Drainage of Cysts.   Any glioma of the spinal cord may be associ-ated with a gliomatous cyst or with a syrinx. It is always desirable to search for these conditions so that, if they are present, they can be drained adequately or evacuated to enhance the decompression. Glioma-tous cysts usually are filled with yellow fluid of a high protein content. The most effective way to eliminate these is to do a longitudinal mye-lotomy and remove as much of the adjacent tumor as possible, leaving a large cavity in contact with the spinal subarachnoid space. Syringo-myelic or hydromyelic cavities associated with gliomas can be evacuated by performance of myelotomy and removal of as much of the tumor as possible. The tumor, however, may not be situated adjacent to the cav-ity. In addition, the communication between the cavity and the subarach-noid space may be kept open by a suture placed between the cavity and the subarachnoid space, acting as a wick [Kirgis-Echols[155] (1949)]. One of us (MacCarty) has also placed one end of a fine polyethylene catheter in the cavity and the other end in the subarachnoid space. This seems to be rather effective.

Removal of Gliomas.   Ependymomas of the filum terminale, as well as a few other rare intramedullary tumors in this area, lend them-selves well to almost complete, if not complete, removal. They present themselves essentially as extramedullary tumors. If the tumor is not too large, the tumor and filum can be removed without injury to the conus and the cauda equina. Of course, many of these neoplasms are large, and either they involve the conus and cauda equina as a result of "seeding" of daughter tumors, so that complete removal is impossible, or they are so intimately bound to the nerve roots or cord substance of the conus (as an epidermoid might be)[4] that total excision is impossible.

Ependymomas situated above the level of the filum terminale are unique in that they can be almost completely, if not occasionally completely, removed. A recent case illustrates what can be accomplished toward removal of an extensive ependymoma of the cervical and thoracic segments of the spinal cord. The neoplasm in question was of particular pathologic interest in that a gliomatous cyst and a syringomyelic cavity were associated with the neoplasm. The gliomatous cyst containing yellow fluid was situated in the posterior part of the upper left side of the cervical cord. Syringomyelia had developed in the upper part of the cervical segment of the cord near the central area of the canal. The neoplasm extended from the upper part of the cervical segment, just below the fourth ventricle, to the fourth thoracic segment. It was removed by performance of suboccipital craniectomy, total cervical laminectomy, and upper thoracic laminectomy. The tumor did not extend to the obex of the fourth ventricle. The contents of the cyst and hydromyelic cavity were evacuated, and the neoplasm was removed by myelotomy extending from the second cervical to the fourth thoracic segments of the spinal cord. The principal neurologic deficits were loss of posterior-column sense and weakness of the upper extremities, particularly the left, and a dissociated sensory defect over the upper part of the trunk and the upper extremities.

After this type of surgical treatment performance of prophylactic tracheotomy is imperative. Assisted respiration for several days or even weeks may be necessary, as it was in this case. Pneumonia may be a severe postoperative complication, but, if these precautions are instituted immediately after the operation, the patient may survive, as did the young woman in the foregoing case.

Because one of us (MacCarty) has never been able to remove an intramedullary tumor above the filum terminale in one piece without interrupting the pseudocapsule, he believes it advisable to irradiate the involved area with the objective of prolonging the time of recurrence.

Spinal Cordectomy.   In rare instances, when useful function of the cord has been completely interrupted by a tumor of that structure, all or a portion of the spinal cord which contains tumor elements can be removed below the cervical segments [MacCarty-Kiefer[187] (1949)]. Obviously, such procedures have limited value and of course should be performed only when complete paraplegia is present and to prevent the tumor from ascending into the cervical segments, producing quadriplegia and death. If a tumor situated in the thoracic segment of the cord has produced spastic paraplegia, the tumor-bearing portion of the spinal cord in this segment can be excised, but to produce flaccidity the remaining distal portion of the cord also can be removed. If it is desired to leave intact a segment of spinal cord which supplies the abdominal musculature, so that this musculature will remain spastic, this can be done. The conus and part of the cauda equina can be removed to produce flaccidity of the lower extremities and bladder. This procedure has been called "selective spinal cordectomy" [MacCarty[186](1954)].

As an example: Excision of an astrocytoma involving the third to the seventh thoracic segments might be carried out from the first to the ninth thoracic segments, and the segment from the ninth to the twelfth thoracic segments could be left intact and the remaining distal portion of the cord excised. There is reason to believe that preservation of some reflex spasm in the abdominal musculature aids the patient in voiding by maintaining some degree of reflex pressure in the abdominal cavity. Thus voiding is aided by the "Credé maneuver" and reflex spasm of the abdominal muscles. The longest segment of spinal cord which one of us (MacCarty) has removed extended from the first thoracic segment through the conus and part of the cauda equina. If it is desired to remove only the tumor-bearing portion of the cord, and spasticity persists, the cauda equina can be destroyed by the intrathecal injection of alcohol as a secondary procedure [Cooper-Hoen[50] (1949); Shelden-Bors[263] (1948)]. Anterior rhizotomy [Munro[198] (1952)] of the cauda equina and selective neurectomies [Bors[22] (1954); Meirowsky and associates[193] (1950)] are other operative measures to produce flaccidity of the lower extremities and bladder.

Secondary Effects of Spinal Cordectomy
and Paraplegia

Paraplegia may be associated with secondary manifestations which can be sufficiently severe to produce complications resulting in death. Dysfunction of the bladder and bowel is always an immediate and permanent source of distress in the paraplegic patient. It is usually desirable to convert spasticity of the bladder to flaccidity. In the male, however, it is necessary to determine the degree of sexual function which is present, because some paraplegic males retain varying degrees of sexual activity which would be abolished by destruction of the cauda equina or conus.

The catabolic effects of paraplegia are profound. They are manifest clinically by osteoporosis, bedsores, and loss of weight. Our investigations have shown evidence of lowered excretion of 17-ketosteroids and corticosteroids, creatinuria, hypoproteinemia, testicular atrophy, decreased hepatic function and metabolic rate, and, in many males, associated gynecomastia [Cooper-Hoen[49] (1949); Cooper and associates (1949[52]), (1950[53])]. It has therefore been our policy to use a high-protein diet and an anticatabolic agent such as testosterone propionate to combat the marked catabolic response associated particularly with acute paraplegia.

Infection of the urinary tract is combated with antibiotic and chemo-therapeutic agents. Transurethral resection of the neck of the bladder has been beneficial in the maintenance of proper evacuation of the bladder, so that in many instances the use of an indwelling catheter becomes unnecessary. Regulation of the bowels can be developed with a proper and consistent program involving the use of an oily laxative agent and enemas.

Enough cannot be said about the important role of the physiatrist in the rehabilitation of paraplegic and quadriplegic patients. Physical medicine can help patients who are paraplegic or even quadriplegic, as a result of accidental injury to the spinal cord or as a result of a tumor of the spinal cord, to lead useful and productive lives.

II

Intramedullary Gliomas of the Spinal Cord and Filum Terminale

Both the brain and the spinal cord have a similar embryologic background, and each is composed essentially of the same cellular elements. Hence, it can be expected that the tumors of both organs will be closely similar. Like tumors of the brain, tumors of the spinal cord can be divided into two complex groups: (1) those which arise from the nervous tissue (neuro-ectodermal or gliomatous tumors); and (2) those which arise from other than nervous tissue (nongliomatous tumors).

The name "gliomatous tumors" or, more conveniently, "gliomas," refers to a large group of tumors of varied gross and histologic appearance. The name includes tumors which originate from the neuroglia itself, those which arise from ependymal cells, and those which arise from nerve cells. Groups which can be recognized are astrocytomas, ependymomas, oligodendrogliomas, subependymal gliomas, and spongioblastomas. To these can be added medulloblastomas and the neuro-astrocytomas, but, since we did not encounter the latter two types in our series of tumors of the spinal cord, we shall not discuss them herein.

Nongliomatous tumors are a mixed group which includes tumors arising from the mesenchymal tissues, such as blood vessels, nerve sheaths, and connective tissue, and tumors originating from developmental defects, such as epidermoids, dermoids, and teratomas. Tumors of nongliomatous origin will be dealt with more extensively in Chapter III.

A special word needs to be said about the malignancy of tumors of nervous tissue. In 1958 Sayre and one of us (Kernohan[148]) wrote, "All tumors of the nervous system are malignant, even if of a low malignancy." It must be emphasized that this statement applies also to tumors

29

originating in the spinal cord and filum terminale, although the factor of malignancy may appear to be less evident. If tumors of the spinal cord are not removed or destroyed completely, they tend to expand and to extend, and in an occasional instance even metastasis develops. The threat to life, especially in respect to tumors located in the lower levels of the spinal cord, is less direct than that of tumors of the brain, but in the more malignant forms and in tumors located in the higher vertebral levels, this particular danger is readily apparent. As will be shown later, life expectancy is limited once a tumor of the spinal cord has developed, although it must be admitted that the life expectancy of a patient who has a tumor of the spinal cord is better than that of one who has a tumor of the brain. Part of the difference in life expectancy comes about because tumors of the spinal cord generally are of a lower degree of malignancy than are tumors of the brain. Moreover, a favorable factor in the case of tumors of the spinal cord is that these lesions generally are more likely to be completely removed, which can result in complete cure of the patient.

SYSTEMS OF CLASSIFICATION

Several schemes for classification of gliomatous tumors were suggested before Bailey and Cushing[16] introduced theirs in 1926. This classification was based upon comparison of the most predominant type of cell found in each type of glioma with the types of cells seen during histogenesis of the normal brain. In this way a name was given to the tumor corresponding to the developing cell which the cells of the tumor were supposed to resemble. The authors admitted, however, that a glioma is only rarely composed of one cellular type. Still, classification on the basis of the most predominant cell type was thought to be possible in most instances.

This classification has been widely accepted, mainly by neurologists and neuropathologists, since it offers a reasonable correlation between the histologic appearance of the tumor and the life expectancy of the patient. At the same time, much criticism was directed at the Bailey and Cushing classification, especially by general pathologists and neuro-anatomists, who pointed out primarily the lack of similarity between the developing embryologic cell and the cells composing most of the very malignant gliomas. They also objected to the complexity of the Bailey and Cushing system. General pathologists were aware that the resemblance of immature tumor cells to histogenetic patterns is hypothetic and is rarely recognized in tumors situated elsewhere in the body than the nervous system. Over the years little has been changed in the Bailey and Cushing classification, although several attempts have been made at modification and simplification of it.

In 1949 one of us (Kernohan) and associates[145] published the results of our studies. An attempt was made at a classification based upon the observation that general pathologists, in dealing with carcinomas situated elsewhere in the body than the nervous system, regard malignant cells as anaplastic modifications of normal mature cells. The idea of this classification is, similarly, founded on the assumption that tumor cells, even of the most rapidly growing gliomas, represent different phases of anaplasia of normal cells, rather than representing undifferentiated cells. The suggested classification is based upon the theory of anaplasia of each of the four adult types of cells present in the central nervous system. The four adult types of gliomatous cells in the normal brain and spinal cord are astrocytes, ependymal cells, oligodendrocytes, and nerve cells. Each of these cells can be the focus for development of a glioma. In the brain the astrocyte is more likely to develop into a tumor than is the ependymal cell; oligodendroglial cells are less likely to give rise to tumors, and nerve cells are only rarely the origins of tumors. The foregoing is true of the spinal cord proper, meaning the cord with the exclusion of the filum terminale.

By the simple process of the application of grades—grade 1 for the least malignant through grade 4 for the most malignant—to tumors arising from each type of cell, a simple classification is designed. This system can be employed relatively easily by pathologists, and it is readily understandable by clinicians, since it defines the degree of malignancy, which aids in the determination of the surgical procedure that is most favorable. It also provides a basis for the prognosis.

Since our study is based on this classification, we shall present more details in association with the descriptions of the several tumor groups.

ASTROCYTOMAS

Astrocytes constitute the major portion of the interstitial tissue of the brain and spinal cord. They have attracted the attention of many workers, and most of our present knowledge is derived from studies by Cajal, Del Rio Hortega, and Penfield.

Astrocytes generally are divided into two groups: fibrous astrocytes and protoplasmatic astrocytes, but a common characteristic of cells of both types is that they appear as relatively small, multipolar, stellate-shaped cells. Fibrous astrocytes are found mainly in the white matter of the brain and spinal cord. They have numerous smooth, thin, fairly straight cellular processes running in all directions from the cell body. These processes branch infrequently, this branching takes place at more acute angles than in the protoplasmatic astrocytes, and they extend to a considerable distance from the cell body. Fibrous astrocytes contain fine fibrilla which extend from one expansion through the cell body to another expansion. These fibrilla can be visualized only by the use of specific stains, such as Mallory's phosphotungstic acid or the Holzer stain. The astrocytic cell body and the processes, but not the fibrilla, can be studied best after specific staining with Cajal's gold chloride and sublimate method.

Protoplasmatic astrocytes, present chiefly in the gray matter of the brain and spinal cord, are characterized by numerous freely branching, relatively short, protoplasmatic processes which radiate from the cell body. These processes are heavier and shorter than are those of the fibrous astrocytes.

The cellular processes of the astrocytes ramify among the nerve cells and in the fiber tracts. A number of the processes are attached to small blood vessels by means of one or several perivascular, footlike structures.

The nucleus of the astrocyte is fairly regular and oval. It is smaller than the ependymal nucleus and is slightly larger than the oglioden-droglial nucleus. The chromatin of the astrocyte is scattered evenly in the nucleus and is moderate to small in amount. The cytoplasm of the astrocyte appears to be slightly granular when subjected to Cajal's gold chloride and sublimate method, and granules of pigment appear to be present, especially in older persons.

Astrocytes are thought to have several specific functions, and some of these are: supporting tissue for the nerve cells and fiber tracts and an intermediate means of nutritional transport. Astrocytes also exhibit swelling and proliferation as reactions to certain types of trauma to the central nervous tissue.

According to Scherer[255] (1940), Abernethy in 1804 was the first to recognize macroscopically tumors of a gliomatous nature. It was Virchow, however, according to many authors, who contributed extensively to knowledge about those tumors. He created the term "glioma," a word which indicates the relationship of certain tumor forms to the neuroglia. At the same time, he divided gliomas into three groups: medullary, fibrous, and telangiectatic. In addition to his work on gliomas, he recognized myxomas and sarcomas of the brain. His description[292] (1864) of sarcomas of the brain corresponds fairly well with modern descriptions of what are now recognized as astrocytomas, grades 3 and 4.

Bailey[12] (1932) credited Golgi (1875) with being the first to insist that the diagnosis of glioma should be dependent upon the presence of star-shaped cells, which now are recognized as astrocytes.

Ribbert[227] in 1918, Strauss and Globus[275] in 1918, and Globus and Strauss[105] in 1925 made early attempts to correlate what was known about tumors of the central nervous system with a histogenetic scheme which described the various stages in the development of the cellular components of the brain and spinal cord. This concept reached a culmination in the classic work of Bailey and Cushing[16] in 1926. In their study they recognized, among other lesions, spongioblastoma multiforme and spongioblastoma unipolare, astroblastoma, and protoplasmatic and fibrillar astrocytomas.

Although this system became widely used, many objections to it have developed and persisted, directed mostly against certain discrepancies having to do with astroblastoma and spongioblastoma multiforme. One of these discrepancies concerned the places which the astroblastoma and glioblastoma multiforme (the spongioblastoma multiforme had been renamed on the ground that the cell did not resemble the histogenetic spongioblast) should occupy in the histogenetic system. The description and classification of the astroblastoma also were attacked because the limits were ill defined and artificial. In their classification of astroblastoma Bailey and Cushing did not adhere closely to histogenetic data; they stressed, rather, a histologic arrangement (a perivascular pattern of the astroblasts around a blood vessel), but included also as a criterion the life history of the tumor. Bailey and Bucy[15] (1930) wrote that the astroblastoma passes over by invisible transformation to become such forms as glioblastoma multiforme, malignant ependymoma, and even astrocytoma. Elvidge, Penfield, and Cone[84] (1937) expressed the opinion that the astroblastoma is histologically and biologically a form between astrocytoma and glioblastoma multiforme.

Variations which the glioblastoma multiforme may manifest constituted another point of considerable discussion, but the general agreement was that the glioblastoma multiforme is of glial origin. In the histogenetic system, however, no cell was known which resembled the abnormal cells of the glioblastoma. Penfield[213] (1931) wrote that in a consideration of this tumor it was difficult to select a single cell type which could be identified with any of the cell types in the spongioblastic series, and this fact made the histogenetic classification of this tumor a problem. Scherer[254] (1940), however, noted that some portions of a glioblastoma multiforme frequently are intermixed with astrocytomatous tissue. He also recognized that the occurrence of pure astrocytomas in the brain is rare, and that the tumors often contain areas which have the structure of a glioblastoma. He concluded that a certain number—the so-called secondary glioblastomas—are dedifferentiated from astrocytes. On the basis of Scherer's study it would appear that at least a certain number of glioblastomas are regarded as more malignant variants of astrocytomas. Canti, Bland, and Russell[43] in 1937 emphasized the point that in tissue cultures the cells of glioblastoma multiforme often come to resemble astrocytes.

An increasing number of pathologists favored the notion that not only astrocytomas and glioblastomas multiforme, but also astroblastomas, represent different degrees of malignancy of the same type of neoplasm.

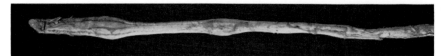

Figure 1. Case 36 in Chapter IV. Spinal cord from a patient who had von Recklinghausen's disease, with four intramedullary tumors (see also Fig. 74).

One of us (Kernohan) and associates[145] (1949) suggested, therefore, that these three tumor groups be regarded as anaplastic variations of the astrocytoma, and that the terms "astroblastoma" and "glioblastoma multiforme" be eliminated. Kernohan and associates applied grades to the tumor forms on the basis of the degree of malignancy: grade 1 for the least malignant to grade 4 for the most malignant form.

The briefly summarized criteria for the various grades of malignancy appear in the original paper by Mabon, Svien, Kernohan, and Craig[185] (1949).

Grade 1 is characterized by relatively normal-appearing astrocytes with no anaplasia.

Grade 2 is characterized by early anaplastic transformation of a small number of cells.

Grade 3 is characterized by moderate anaplastic transformation of roughly half of the cells. Mitotic figures are present; the average is one in each field under the high-power objective.

Grade 4 is characterized by marked anaplastic transformation of most of the cells; mitotic figures are abundant, averaging 4 to 5 in every field under the high-power objective.

Gross Findings.   Most intramedullary tumors of the spinal cord present themselves as fusiform swellings of the spinal cord (Fig. 1).* Often these swellings cause obliteration of the subdural space. In a minority of cases the tumor reaches the surface of the cord, but most often it is completely surrounded by more or less normal but somewhat compressed tissue. The consistency appears mostly to be rather firm and fibrous, but in some descriptions the consistency is said to be gelatinous (as a result of edema) or friable. The outer and cut surfaces often are somewhat granular. The color as described in reports of gross lesions varies from gray and yellow to beefy red, and apparently is influenced by the content of blood and by hemorrhages, edema, and degeneration. In slightly more than a third of cases cysts are described; rather often these cysts are filled with a golden-yellow gelatinous fluid which clots easily. The cysts are present in the substance of the tumor, as well as at the borderline of the lesion with relatively normal tissues. Some cysts in the latter location are not invariably cysts of the tumor itself, but are syringomyelic cavities (see Chapter IV). It is characteristic of the lower grade astrocytomas that generally they do not possess a clear line of

* See Figure 74 and case 36 in Chapter IV.

demarcation, an occurrence which limits the effectiveness of the surgeon because it often prevents him from removing the tumor completely.

Only a few astrocytomas originate from the filum terminale. When they do, they appear grossly as either smooth swellings of this structure or as a round bulging mass attached to it.

Histologic Aspects

Grade 1 Astrocytoma. Two types of astrocytes are known: fibrillar and protoplasmatic. Two types of astrocytomas also are generally recognized: fibrillar or fibrous, and protoplasmatic. Development of the protoplasmatic astrocytoma in the brain or in the spinal cord is fairly uncommon.

The grade 1 fibrillar astrocytoma is composed essentially of an increased number of relatively normal-appearing fibrillar astrocytes (Fig. 2) which generally also have a normal-appearing nucleus. The nuclei are small to medium (Fig. 3) and are mostly round to oval, but occasionally are more spindle shaped or even somewhat irregular in outline. There is little or no pleomorphism and giant nuclei are not present; very rarely a multinucleated cell can be found. The nuclei usually appear to be located in the center of the cell body, but an eccentric location is sometimes observed. There is always a distinct nuclear outline. The chromatin content is variable; as a rule it is moderate, but sometimes it is heavier; frequently the chromatin is structureless and smooth, but occasionally it may appear to be finely or even coarsely granular. In nearly all instances the chromatin is evenly distributed over the karyo-

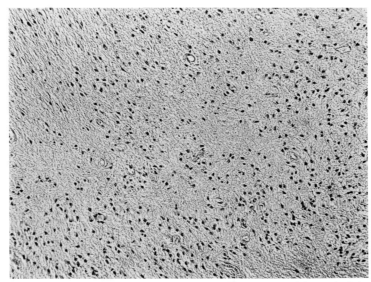

Figure 2. A grade 1 astrocytoma, fibrillary type, with marked increase and compactness of the glial fibrils (hematoxylin and eosin; × 150)

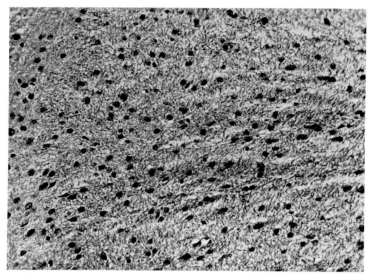

Figure 3. A grade 1 astrocytoma. The nuclei are evenly distributed and moderately sized. There is no pleomorphism or hyperchromatism (hematoxylin and eosin; × 300).

plasm, but in some tumors the nuclei tend to have a more vesicular appearance. An occasional nucleus may have a more septated aspect which seems to be the result of several vacuoles in the karyoplasm; otherwise, nuclear vacuoles are considered to be fairly rare in the lower grade astrocytomas. Nucleoli are fairly uncommon, although this factor varied in the several tumors in our series. Mitosis is absent. A few inclusion bodies were found in some tumors.

The nuclei are surrounded by a small amount of protoplasm forming the small, often triangular or polygonal, stellate-shaped cell body of the fibrillar astrocyte. From this cell body several cellular processes are seen running in all directions. These cellular processes taper fairly rapidly to become long, slender filaments. Stained with hematoxylin and eosin, these processes are difficult to follow, since they intermingle in the intercellular matrix. Infrequently all the cellular details and the cellular outlines of the fibrillar astrocytes can be discerned, but they are mostly vague and difficult to distinguish from the intercellular substance. Visualization is simplified by use of several of the special staining technics, such as Cajal's gold chloride and sublimate method, the Mallory phosphotungstic acid stain, or the Holzer stain. Some of the processes are seen to attach themselves to the wall of an adjacent blood vessel, but usually this feature is not observed. The cytoplasm appears at times to contain fine, densely-packed granules, but sometimes it has a more nearly foamy appearance. Intracellular vacuoles are found only rarely.

Astrocytomas do not have a characteristic architecture. The cellular density of the grade 1 astrocytomas exceeds only slightly the normal density of tissue of the spinal cord. Neoplastic cells for the most part are fairly evenly distributed throughout the tumor. Recognition of the entity as a neoplasm is facilitated by the increased density (sometimes marked) of neuroglial fibrils (Fig. 2) and by the absence or decrease of normal structures such as myelin sheaths, axis cylinders, oligodendrocytes, and ganglion cells in the central area of the tumor. At the edges of the tumor there is often an intermingling of the neoplastic structures and the pre-existent, but now distorted, nervous tissue. This results mostly in a broad zone of transition, and there is no sharp line of demarcation.

The matrix or intercellular substance of the fibrous astrocytoma is composed of a myriad of dense, intertwining processes, nearly all of which stain specifically for neuroglial fibrils when specific stains are used. The number apparently is independent of the number of nuclei present, since in most instances in our series only a relatively small number of nuclei were present in an extremely dense neuroglial network.

The fibrils are not always densely packed, and occasionally they are separated by many irregular-shaped intercellular spaces, vacuoles, or microcysts of varying size (Fig. 4). Occasionally these vacuoles merge into larger cysts. The content of the vacuoles does not stain with the ordinary stains, but the larger cysts sometimes contain material which stains faint pink with eosin. Most probably these spaces are the results of edema of the tumor, although, according to some authors [Elvidge and associates[84] (1937)], they also may be produced or enlarged by degeneration within or at the borderline of the tumor. In some cases the formation of vacuoles is so advanced that only a spongy network of tumor tissue is left, and the astrocytic nuclei are found at the center of the junctions of the meshes

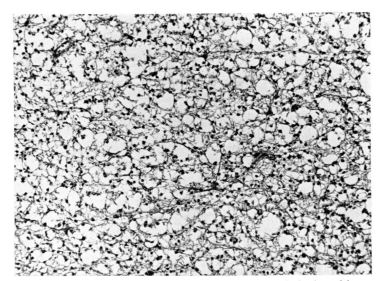

Figure 4. An edematous grade 1 astrocytoma. Irregularly shaped inter-cellular spaces and vacuoles (hematoxylin and eosin; × 150).

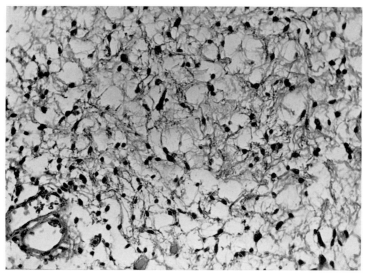

Figure 5. A grade 1 astrocytoma. Marked intercellular edema with the nuclei located at the junction of the meshes (hematoxylin and eosin; × 300).

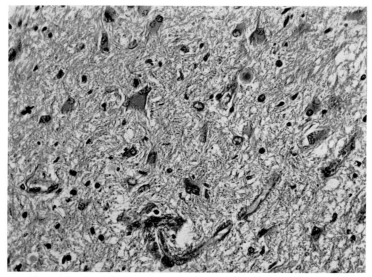

Figure 6. A grade 1 astrocytoma in case 13, Chapter IV. A group of gemistocytic astrocytes are seen in an otherwise fibrillary astrocytoma (hematoxylin and eosin; × 300).

(Fig. 5). It appears that the fibrillary density in these circumstances is less than the average which otherwise is seen.

In our series a few astrocytes were found which had a swollen, clear, pink-staining cell body (Fig. 6). It appeared that these cells had fewer and shorter processes than are usually seen. These so-called gemistocytic

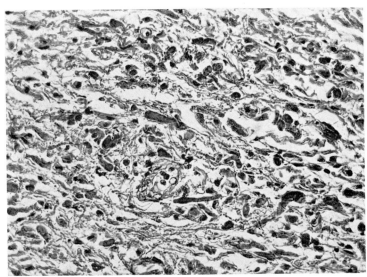

Figure 7. A grade 1 astrocytoma, showing Rosenthal fibers in varying sizes and shapes (hematoxylin and eosin; × 300).

astrocytes are a well-recognized variant of fibrillary astrocytes. We found,
however, no tumor in our series in which such cells were dominant; in
only a few areas of several tumors they were intermingled with the usual
fibrillar astrocytomatous cells. In a few other tumors we found that the
tumor cells had a more elongated aspect, with fairly thick, more slowly
tapering processes extending from both ends of the cells. The nuclei of
these cells were more spindle shaped, and were located centrally in the
cell. Only an occasional tumor was completely composed of such cells,
but this type of cell arrangement was seen a few times in combination
with the other patterns.

We had no example of a protoplasmatic astrocytoma in our series of
grade 1 tumors.

In about 10 per cent of the grade 1 astrocytomas, so-called Rosenthal
fibers (Fig. 7) were found. These are most often carrot-shaped, sometimes
tortuous, homogeneous, deeply purple, eosinophilic-staining masses of
unknown significance. Sometimes they are cut transversely, and then
they appear as round bodies mostly homogeneous but sometimes presenting a vague indication of an internal lamellar structure. In our series
an occasional one appeared to contain a nucleus. They also occur in
the presence of various other conditions (see syringomyelia), and generally are regarded as degeneration of the neuroglial cells.

Calcification of blood vessels, as well as interstitial calcification and
calcification in the tumor cells, sometimes is found.

Most grade 1 astrocytomas contained relatively few blood vessels, but
a few tumors exhibited a moderate increase. As a rule there is little or
no tendency toward endothelial or adventitial proliferation, but hyalin-

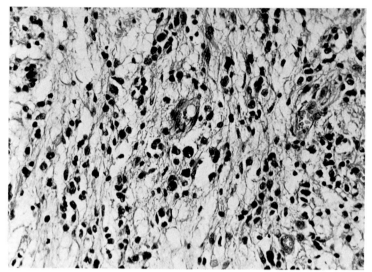

Figure 8. A grade 2 astrocytoma, showing moderate pleomorphism
and hyperchromatism of the nuclei (hematoxylin and eosin; × 300).

ization of the walls of the vessels is not too uncommon. Sometimes a
cuff of lymphocytes is seen around a blood vessel.

Grade 2 Astrocytoma.   Most of the cells in tumors of this grade can
be recognized easily as astrocytes which are not dissimilar to those of
grade 1 astrocytomas. The remaining cells, however, show early anaplastic transformation (Fig. 8) which consists of a slight-to-moderately increased pleomorphism of the nuclei and cells. The nuclei have a general
tendency to be increased in size, and their form is less regular than that
of normal cells. The nuclei stain with a moderately irregular intensity
which is the result of the heavier chromatin content of some of them.
Occasionally, the chromatin appears as coarsely irregular granules, and
these sometimes are scattered unevenly through the karyoplasm. Nuclear
vacuoles sometimes are present, and only a few inclusion bodies may be
found. Mitotic figures are absent, but a few large cells, almost approach-
ing giant cells, and multinucleated cells were present in a few of the
cases. Slight pleomorphism is seen in some of the cell bodies, and the
processes of the cells can be impregnated readily with Cajal's gold
chloride and sublimate method. Glial fibrils, however, appear to be
fewer, and many of the processes are not so long and delicate as in
tumors of grade 1 malignancy.

A specific quality of grade 2 astrocytomas consists of a focal, often
multiple, or a generalized increased cellularity (Fig. 9). Formation of
both cysts and zones of necrosis may be present, but is very uncommon.
As is true of grade 1 tumors, there are no recognizable architectural
patterns. The zone of transition to the normal surrounding tissue generally is regarded as somewhat narrower than that found in grade 1

astrocytomas. Another feature characteristic of increased malignancy is the slight proliferation of the blood vessels, and as a consequence grade 2 astrocytomas tend to have a slight-to-moderately increased vascularity. Proliferation of the endothelial cells lining the blood vessels is sometimes seen, but as a rule this change is not impressive. Hyaline thickening of walls of vessels was prominent in a few tumors, and was present to a lesser degree in several others.

Cells loaded with coarse, brown, iron-containing granules were found in a few tumors. They were regarded as representing old hemorrhage.

In some grade 2 astrocytomas a few cell groups were found which were interpreted as being either ependymal cells or oligodendroglial cells. The areas of the latter were not so impressive as in the ependymomas. It might well be that the ependymal cells are derived from the area of the central canal, and are not integral parts of the tumor, but are simply included in the tumor much as ganglion cells sometimes are found embedded in a tumor.

In one of the tumors the astrocytes appeared to be swollen, and contained a clear pink cytoplasm. The nucleus was found chiefly in the periphery of the cell. These cells had several fairly coarse, thick but short processes. This tumor was judged to be a gemistocytic astrocytoma, although it contained areas which had the architecture of a fibrillar astrocytoma. In several other tumors small areas containing gemistocytic astrocytes were found.

We found no example in our series of a protoplasmatic astrocytoma,

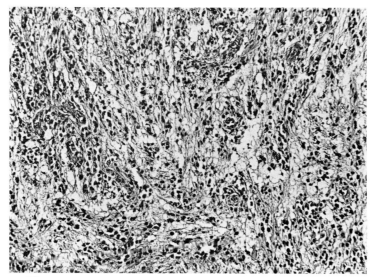

Figure 9. A grade 2 astrocytoma, same case as in Figure 8, showing increased cellularity and slight intercellular edema (hematoxylin and eosin; × 150).

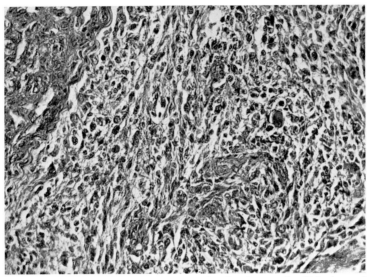

Figure 10. A grade 3 astrocytoma, showing increased cellularity and pleomorphism. Note also the marked swelling and proliferation of the endothelial cells of the blood vessels (hematoxylin and eosin; × 250).

grade 2, although small groups of cells characteristic of such a tumor occasionally were found.

Grade 3 Astrocytoma.   A great number of cells in the grade 3 astrocytoma still can be identified easily as astrocytes, although only a small number of them are essentially normal. The grade 3 astrocytoma presents an increase in cellularity (Fig. 10), but the degree is variable. The nuclei of many cells are increased in size; the form of the nuclei is more variable than in the previous types. A number of them are irregular in outline and are fairly large, and could be designated as "giant nuclei." A striking difference in the nuclear chromatin content becomes even more apparent in this type. Some nuclei contain a normal, moderate amount of chromatin, but a larger number are markedly hyperchromatic and stand out clearly. Such hyperchromatic nuclei are chiefly ones that are enlarged and irregular in form. The chromatin often becomes condensed into large, irregular-staining clumps, giving the nucleus a bizarre aspect. This type of tumor exhibits an increasing tendency toward multinucleated cells. The number of mitotic figures is somewhat variable, but generally it is not very high.

The cell body of the grade 3 astrocytoma also is rather pleomorphic. Around some of the nuclei only traces of cytoplasm can be distinguished, whereas others have a marked amount. In some tumors we found areas consisting of a number of gemistocytic astrocytes. The cellular outlines, when distinguishable, often are irregular. As a rule the cellular processes are heavier, shorter, and less numerous, and may be even lacking in the case of the more anaplastic cells. Those cells which can be recognized may be multipolar, bipolar, or even unipolar; others appear to be polygonal or round or oval. Treatment with special stains shows that a number of the cells still can be impregnated when Cajal's method is used and that there are a varying number of neuroglial fibrils remaining. The grade 3 astrocytoma, however, has less of an affinity for the stains than do astrocytomas of lower grades, but generally it also has fewer fibrils. The amount of intercellular fibrils appears to be somewhat related to the number of fairly normal-appearing astrocytes which are present, and consequently it is considerably less than in astrocytomas of grade 1 and grade 2. A varying degree of intercellular edema is seen, but there is practically no tendency toward the formation of cysts. The tumor cells do not give indication of any type of arrangement except that of palisading around small foci of necrosis. We did not see any Rosenthal fibers in this type of tumor.

Almost all the tumors of this type showed at least a moderate increase in vascularity, and changes in blood vessels were encountered rather frequently. Most marked is the proliferation of the endothelial cells lining the blood vessels (Fig. 11), but proliferation of the adventitial cells is not uncommon. Mitosis of the endothelial cells sometimes is seen. The vascular lumina may be narrowed or occasionally even occluded; if the latter has occurred, it may be responsible, at least in part, for the increased tendency toward foci of necrosis and degeneration.

The transitional zone between normal and neoplastic tissue is far more sharply defined than it is in tumors of lower grades. The surrounding non-neoplastic tissue sometimes exhibits a slight gliosis which should

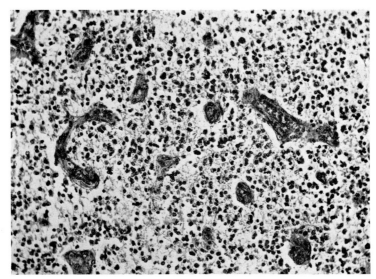

Figure 11. A grade 3 astrocytoma, showing increased vascularity with swelling and proliferation of the endothelial cells (hematoxylin and eosin; × 200).

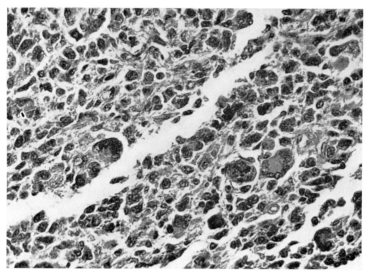

Figure 12. A grade 4 astrocytoma described in case 17, Chapter IV, showing very marked pleomorphism with giant nuclei and multinucleated cells and pronounced hyperchromatism. Note the tripolar mitosis (hematoxylin and eosin; × 375).

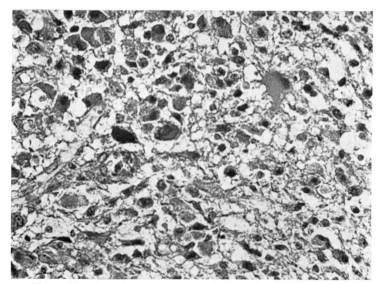

Figure 13. A grade 4 astrocytoma in case 5, Chapters II and IV, showing the variable sizes and shapes of the astrocytes. Most of the astrocytes still have recognizable cellular processes (hematoxylin and eosin; × 375).

be distinguished from the neoplastic cells and in which gemistocytic astrocytes can be dominant. These cells probably are reactive to the damage of the tissue of the spinal cord.

Grade 4 Astrocytoma.   The line of gradually increasing anaplastic changes culminates in the astrocytoma of this grade, and it ranges among the most malignant-appearing tumor forms occurring in the human body. Cellularity is greatly increased, but there is a decrease in the number of relatively normal-appearing astrocytes. There is not only a relative but also an absolute increase in the number of highly malignant anaplastic cells (Fig. 12), which often have huge, irregular, bizarre giant nuclei which contain irregular masses of chromatin. Hyperchromatism often is impressive, and multinucleated giant cells are fairly frequent in some tumors. The appearance of the cellular form, if this is recognizable, is very variable (Fig. 13), and often an admixture of many shapes and sizes is seen. Gemistocytic astrocytes are present very infrequently. The number of mitotic figures is markedly increased, and among them are a fair number of abnormal forms. As in the types previously considered herein, there is no architectural pattern; to the contrary, grade 4 astrocytomas are impressive by virtue of their very disorganized appearance. The only arrangement which exists is a palisading of the cells around areas of necrosis (Fig. 14).

The increased vascularity is evident despite a partial or even complete occlusion of the vascular lumina by proliferation and swelling of endothelial and adventitial cells. Often the proliferative vascular structures stand out in a histologic section because of their different nuclear structure, which is less hyperchromatic than that of the astrocytes. Mitosis in these vascular lesions is not uncommon.

Areas of necrosis frequently are encountered; they are more extensive than in grade 3 astrocytomas, but they appear to be somewhat less im-

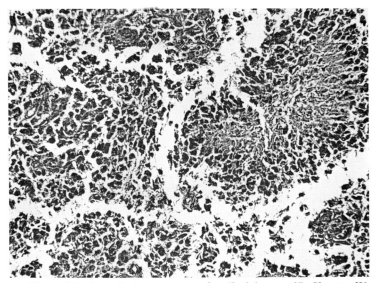

Figure 14. A grade 4 astrocytoma described in case 17, Chapter IV, showing one area of necrosis and indication of palisading of the astrocytes around the area (hematoxylin and eosin; × 175).

pressive than in grade 4 astrocytomas of the brain. The degree of fibrillary development decreases according to the number of normal-appearing cells, and in this grade of lesion fibrillary development is minimal. The degree of intercellular edema is variable, and can be extensive, but formation of cysts is uncommon.

Microscopically, the line of demarcation between the tumor and the surrounding tissue often is quite sharp.

Report of Cases of Astrocytomas

Case 1

A 21-year-old woman experienced pain between and under the shoulder blades 10 months before she came to the Mayo Clinic in 1958. This pain had disappeared within about a week, but 5 months later it recurred. The pain then became constant and worse, especially at night. It was accompanied by tingling and numbness in the right fourth and fifth fingers. The patient also experienced an episode of numbness of the right side of the chest and abdomen. This subsided, as did some of the numbness in the right extremity, but it returned again shortly afterward. The patient also said she noticed a sensation of "electricity" in her spinal column when she coughed or bent her head forward. The history indicated that the patient had had encephalitis at the age of 14 years and had sustained crushing of the first and second lumbar vertebrae in a fall from a horse at the age of 17 years.

Results of the physical examination were essentially negative. Objectively, the area of numbness appeared to be causing minimal disturbance and was spotty. The neurologic examination disclosed nothing of significance.

A roentgenogram of the spinal column revealed an old fracture of the first and second lumbar vertebrae and an unusual reversal of the cervical lordotic curve between the fourth and fifth cervical vertebrae. Spinal puncture was done; the only significant finding was a protein content of 90 mg. per 100 cc. of fluid, with only 2 cells per cubic millimeter. A myelogram made with Pantopaque as a contrast medium was interpreted as showing an intradural but extramedullary tumor, 5 by 1.5 cm., on the right side opposite the sixth and seventh cervical vertebrae.

Laminectomy was then performed; the sixth and seventh cervical and the first thoracic laminae were removed. After the dura had been opened the surgeon was surprised to see a typical grayish astrocytoma in the dorsal column on the right side. A portion of the tumor was removed, and an attempt was made to establish a line of demarcation between the tumor and normal tissue, but this appeared to be impossible. Therefore, the dura was tacked laterally, the dentate ligaments were cut, and polyethylene was placed over the dural defect. An elliptic incision was made in the polyethylene over the extruding tumor in the hope that the tumor would extend itself into the muscle rather than intraspinally.

Histologically, the tumor was classified as a grade 1 astrocytoma.

The postoperative course was uneventful, and the patient's objective complaints abated slightly. During the postoperative course the patient received 16 sessions of cobalt 60 irradiation over the lower cervical and high thoracic areas of the spinal cord. After this course fever of undetermined origin developed, but neutropenia was noted. This condition cleared slowly, and the patient was dismissed.

Twenty-one months after the operation the patient reported that she still noticed some degree of tingling in the right third, fourth, and fifth fingers and a sensation of numbness over the chest. Occasionally, she experienced a sharp pain in the back, but otherwise she considered herself to be in good health.

Case 2

A woman 21 years old said that at the age of 14 years, without apparent cause, she had begun to experience difficulty in maintaining her equilibrium. Foot drop had appeared on the left. This was soon followed by complete spastic paralysis in the lower extremities. There was no change in sensation. This condition had cleared in 1½ years, and she had remained completely well during the ensuing 1½ years. She had attended school, and had played tennis and could dance. Then she had begun to notice difficulty in descending stairs, as well as apparent loss of strength in both legs. Complete loss of sensation below the level of the seventh rib developed, and control of the vesical and anal sphincters was lost. She encountered difficulty in the use of the arms, and she complained of some degree of pain in the neck.

Examination revealed complete spastic paralysis of the legs, with marked ankle clonus. All the reflexes were exaggerated, and Babinski's sign was elicited bilaterally. Cutaneous sensibility was completely lost up to the level of the third thoracic vertebra.

Roentgenologic examination of the thoracic and cervical areas of the spinal column disclosed nothing of significance.

Laminectomy was performed (in 1917) by removal of the laminae of the sixth and seventh cervical and the first three thoracic vertebrae. The dura was found to bulge to a marked degree; when it was opened the spinal cord extruded through the incision. After a longitudinal incision was made in the spinal cord a brown, cystic, necrotic mass was seen. A clear line of demarcation was not evident, but as much as possible of the tumor was removed. The dura was left open, and the exposed portion of spinal cord was covered with animal membrane.

Histologically, the tumor was diagnosed as a grade 1 fibrillar astrocytoma.

The postoperative course was uneventful, but there was no change in the neurologic condition except that the disturbances in the patient's arms cleared completely. Through the years after the operation we received many letters from her. Her condition remained completely stationary and she was able to make a living by sewing. The last letter we received from her was written 31 years (in 1948) after the operation. At that time the only additional development consisted of sores and decubital ulcers. After 1948 we were unable to locate the patient.

Case 3

Some 23 months before he underwent surgery for a tumor of the spinal cord in 1955, a man 67 years old noted the onset of a dead, dull, burning pain in the lower part of the back, right hip, and the posterior aspect of the right thigh, leg, and foot. The pain was associated with numbness over some areas; at first it could be relieved by exercise, the local application of heat, or by his lying down. During the ensuing months there was an insidious increase in the difficulties, and the pain extended into the right lower quadrant of the abdomen and into the right testicle. It was also reported that the size and force of the urinary stream decreased, and for this reason prostatectomy was performed. This operation had no effect upon the pain. Six months after the onset of pain, orthopedic and neurologic consultation was sought, but no positive observations were made at this time. During the next 5 months the patient received physical therapy, injections of vitamin B_{12}, cortisone, histamine, and diathermy. All these measures were without success. Nearly a year after the onset of the pain an electromyogram demonstrated changes consistent with pressure on the sciatic nerve. Laminectomy was performed. A ruptured intervertebral disk in the right fourth intervertebral space was found and removed.

During the next 6 months physiotherapy was continued. A second electromyogram made at the end of this period was reported to show changes similar to those in the first one, and a second laminectomy was done. It was found that the fourth articular facet lay loose; this was removed. It was also noted that the fifth nerve root was compressed by bone and scar tissue; the foramen therefore was enlarged. Since the root had been traumatized and the scar tissue was extremely dense, the fifth posterior root was dissected out and cut.

Instead of reporting relief, the patient complained that his pain had been aggravated; 2 months after the last surgical treatment and 20 months after the onset of the ailment he noticed that he also experienced pain at night and that exercise failed to bring relief of the pain.

When the patient was seen here, he was experiencing the pain as described, but he also complained of weakness of the right foot and numbness of the right big toe. There was no weakness on the left side.

Slight loss of muscle strength was noted in both lower legs, and −1 anesthesia and −4 analgesia were demonstrated in the distal half of the right lower leg. Routine roentgenologic examination of the lumbar portion of the spinal column showed nothing abnormal except the signs of the previous laminectomies. Lumbar puncture was done; the only noteworthy finding was an elevated protein content 300 mg. per 100 cc.) of the cerebrospinal fluid.

A third bilateral laminectomy was done. At the right side a large intraspinal protrusion of the lumbosacral disk was found and was removed. At the fourth lumbar interspace a ridge of bone, originating from the body of the fifth lumbar vertebra and projecting against the dura and the fifth lumbar root, was noted and was removed.

Postoperatively the patient received cortisone. Some days after the operation a blister developed on the right toe, which was anesthetic. It appeared that the patient had obtained no relief of his pain. Sympathetic block was done, but it produced no relief of the pain. About a month after the operation lumbar puncture was repeated; the protein content of the cerebrospinal fluid at this time was 400 mg. per 100 cc. A myelogram with Pantopaque as the contrast medium was made at this time. It demonstrated a partially obstructing lesion at the level of the second and third dorsal vertebrae.

Laminectomy was then performed at the level of the second and third thoracic vertebrae. After the dura had been opened the spinal cord appeared to be whiter and broader than normal. The cord was incised; a tumor mass was found which had the grayish, firm appearance of an astrocytoma. Biopsy of a section of the tumor was reported to show a grade 2 astrocytoma. Because of the intractable pain which had caused the patient to seek relief at the Mayo Clinic and because it was judged to be impossible to remove enough of the tumor to relieve the pain, left anterolateral tractotomy was done. The postoperative period was uneventful, although complete relief of the pain was not achieved. Cobalt 60 irradiation therapy was started, but this aggravated the pain so much that it was stopped. During this time the patient also had temporary retention of urine which cleared without specific treatment. About a month after he had returned to his home the patient received additional therapy with cobalt 60.

In follow-up studies a note was received which mentioned that the patient had died 14 months after the last operation for tumor of the spinal cord. The cause of death was not given.

Case 4

A girl 15 years old had noted, about 2 months before operative treatment in 1948, that her left lower leg became difficult to use and seemed to drag. At night she was sometimes awakened by pain in both shoulder blades. She was admitted to the local hospital; 6 days after the onset of the pain lumbar puncture was performed. Within a few hours complete paralysis of the lower extremities developed, and retention of urine and cessation of intestinal function supervened. Shortly after this she was found to be completely anesthetic below the level of the clavicles. Retention of urine and cessation of intestinal function were alleviated, but 2½ weeks after onset of the pain a sharp, radiating pain developed around the right side of her chest to the midline of the sternum at the level of the right nipple. This pain subsided spontaneously 3 weeks later. Lumbar puncture was repeated; complete block in the circulation of the cerebrospinal fluid was found. When the patient returned to her home, decubital ulcers developed over the sacrum, and she was referred to the Mayo Clinic.

Examination revealed complete flaccid paralysis of the muscles of the abdominal wall and legs and a slight weakness bilaterally in the hypothenar and interossei muscles. Complete anesthesia for all modalities was demonstrated from the clavicles down to and including the mesial sides of the arms. The tendon reflexes in the arms were slightly increased, but those in the legs were absent.

A roentgenogram of the spinal column revealed slight scoliosis.

Bilateral laminectomy was done by removal of the laminae of the first, second, and third dorsal vertebrae. After the dura had been opened a lesion was found in the left side of the cord; this lesion had destroyed the cord for a distance of an inch. The major portion of the tumor was removed. At the end of the operation the dura was left open. Histologically the tumor proved to be a grade 3 astrocytoma.

The postoperative period was difficult, marked by spiking temperature of as high as 106° F. The patient was treated with antibiotic agents, but despite this, evidence of a septic state persisted for several days. On the eleventh postoperative day it was noted that the wound was gaping over a small portion; resuturing was necessary because of a hematoma. The bedsores healed while the patient was in the hospital.

At the time the patient was dismissed there was no function of the spinal cord below the level of the seventh cervical vertebra.

Approximately 3 months after the operation a letter was received in which it was said that the patient had died. Necropsy was reported to have disclosed that the tumor had extended upward to the base of the brain.

Case 5

A man 27 years old in military service had noted, in 1946, 4 weeks prior to the first of several operations he underwent, numbness extending from the left lower thoracic area to the sacro-iliac region and from the midline in the back to the midline on the abdomen. Examination 3 weeks after the onset of the numbness revealed that sensation of pain was diminished in the left lower extremity. The Babinski sign was elicited on the left, but abdominal reflexes were absent. Roentgenograms showed alternate increased densities of the margins of the bodies of the vertebrae from the fifth through the tenth thoracic vertebrae. At lumbar puncture the initial pressure was 240 cm. of water, but the Queckenstedt procedure demonstrated no abnormality. A myelogram revealed a filling defect at the level of the eighth and ninth thoracic vertebrae. Laminectomy, however, did not reveal a tumor. After receiving a course of roentgen-ray therapy the patient was dismissed. He said there had been a slight limp in the left leg at the time of dismissal.

During the next 10 months there was a progressive loss of motor and sensory functions in the left lower extremity. Examination at the end of that time demonstrated anesthesia and analgesia extending from the sixth dorsal vertebra caudad, and to the left more than to the right, and atrophy of the left lower leg with hyperactive tendon reflexes. Babinski's sign was elicited on the left, grade 4+; and on the right, grade 1+. There was a marked limp in the left leg.

A myelogram revealed narrowing of the spinal canal at the second and third thoracic vertebrae, but a block could not be demonstrated. Twenty sessions of roentgen-ray irradiation were conducted at this time.

Four months later the patient became confined to a wheelchair, and a month later control of the sphincters of the bladder and bowel was lost.

Two months later the patient was seen at the Mayo Clinic and was found to be completely paraplegic below the level of the fourth thoracic vertebra. He was completely anesthetic from the line of the nipples downward. The tendon reflexes in the legs were still exaggerated, and Babinski's sign was elicited bilaterally.

Laminectomy was done in 1948; the laminae of the seventh cervical and the first, second, and third thoracic vertebrae were removed. An elongated, fusiform enlargement of the spinal cord below the level of the first thoracic segment was found. The dorsal columns were split, and a grayish-white tumor, which contained a small cyst, was encountered. The tumor obviously was intermingled with the substance of the spinal cord except around the area of the cyst. Biopsy of a specimen of tissue from the tumor showed it to be a grade 3 astrocytoma. The dura was left open.

After the operation the patient was febrile for several days. After the sutures were removed dehiscence of the wound occurred, but the wound healed after the patient went home. While the patient was at home several decubital ulcers developed. When he returned 4 weeks later no essential change was noted in the neurologic status.

Extensive treatment for the decubital ulcers was instituted, and blood was administered several times for anemia. After this problem had been managed, cordectomy was performed. It was carried from the conus up to the seventh cervical vertebra and was done in two stages. In several areas of the tumor present in the operative specimen malignancy of grade 4 was detected. During the next months several decubital ulcers developed.

Gradually, in the ensuing months, anesthesia extended over the medial sides of both arms, and weakness which ranged as far as paralysis was noted in several muscles of the left arm.

In 1949, 3 years after the onset of the disease process, the patient displayed evidence of intracranial involvement as manifested by nausea, vomiting, and conjugate weakness of the eyes. The patient died 3 weeks after he was last admitted to the Mayo Clinic. Death was caused by progressive cerebral involvement. The observations made at necropsy will be discussed in Chapter IV (case 5).

Clinical Analysis.   Before a detailed description of the clinical data of this series of cases is attempted, it must be emphasized that this study embraces a period of 45 years. At first thought this long span may appear to be advantageous, and to some extent this is true, since the condition of several patients was followed for a long time, with the result that the effect of therapy could be appraised. On the other hand, however, many changes in medicine and surgery occurred during the same span, such as improvement in diagnostic and surgical technics, the introduction of chemotherapy and antibiotic agents, and the like, which have influenced so greatly the clinical course of the disease in question that now it is impossible to form absolute conclusions, over so many years, concerning such factors as the life history of the patient, pre-operative and postoperative periods, and the mortality rate in the face of so many constantly changing factors.

It is judged, however, that even when these factors are taken into consideration, careful study of the clinical data contributes better knowledge and understanding of the behavior of intramedullary tumors of the spinal cord, and, with this judgment in mind, we have attempted a review of the histories. In the appendix is a summary of the main findings among individual patients.

The total number of astrocytomas was 86. Forty-five were classified as grade 1, 21 as grade 2, 15 as grade 3, and five as grade 4. With the exception of six lesions, all were found in the medulla spinalis. It is also clear that astrocytomas are the most common tumors of the spinal cord. Of the six found in the filum terminale two were grade 1, one was grade 2, and three were grade 3.

It is evident that astrocytoma of the filum terminale is rare. It accounts for only 7 per cent of all astrocytomas of the spinal cord. It also can be pointed out, on the basis of these data, that astrocytomas of the spinal cord generally are less malignant in histologic appearance than are astrocytomas of the brain: 52 per cent were grade 1, 24 per cent were grade 2, 18 per cent were grade 3, and 6 per cent were grade 4, whereas, according to Sayre and one of us [Kernohan[147] (1952)], grades 3 and 4 astrocytomas of the brain constitute more than 90 per cent of all gliomas in elderly patients.

Age.   The average age of the patients at the time of operation (Table 9) for a grade 1 lesion was 35 years; among those who had grade 2 lesions it was 38 years and 7 months; among those who had grade 3 lesions it was 30 years and 2 months; and among those who had grade 4 tumors it was 23 years and 5 months. On the basis of this it could be suggested that there is a tendency for the more malignant tumors to occur in the younger age group. The value of this observation is limited, since some of the groups in our series are rather small. Hence, any conclusions drawn therefrom cannot be regarded as entirely valid. The youngest patient among those who had astrocytomas was 16 months, and the oldest was 68 years. As can be seen in Table 10, nearly two thirds (62 per cent) of all the tumors were found while the patients were in the third, fourth, and fifth decades of life, but otherwise there was no predominance of occurrence of the lesions in any specific age group. In Figure 15 curves have been plotted for the age of patients at the time of occurrence of several types of gliomas, neurilemmomas, and meningiomas, and comparison indicates that the curves are fairly similar.

Table 9. *Average Age and Sex of Patients: 86 Intramedullary Astrocytomas, Grades 1 to 4*

Astro-cytomas, Location	Histopathologic Grade																Totals
	1				2				3				4				
	Pa-tients, No.	Average Age, Yr.	Male	Fem.	Pa-tients, No.	Average Age, Yr.	Male	Fem.	Pa-tients No.	Average Age, Yr.	Male	Fem.	Pa-tients, No.	Average Age, Yr.	Male	Fem.	
Total group	45	35	25	20	21	38 7/12	13	8	15	30 2/12	8	7	5	23 5/12	2	3	86
Spinal cord	43	35 1/12	25	18	20	39 4/12	12	8	12	30 1/12	7	5	5	23 5/12	2	3	80
Filum terminale	2	34	–	2	1	23	1	–	3	30 8/12	1	2	–	–	–	–	6

Table 10. *Incidence of 86 Intramedullary Astrocytomas Based Upon Decades of Life of Patients*

Decade	Grade				Total	
	1	2	3	4	No.	Per Cent
0 – 9	5	1	1	1	8	9.4
10 – 19	1	3	2	1	7	8.1
20 – 29	12	4	5	1	22	25.6
30 – 39	8	3	2	2	15	17.3
40 – 49	11	3	3		17	19.7
50 – 59	4	3	2		9	10.5
60 – 69	4	4			8	9.4
Total	45	21	15	5	86	100.0

Sex. Of the 86 astrocytomas, 48 were found in males and 38 in females. Reports in the literature indicate that the occurrence of astrocytomas has a slight predominance among males; this was reflected also in our series. Among those who had tumors of the filum terminale were four females and two males; this group is too small to be of any statistical value.

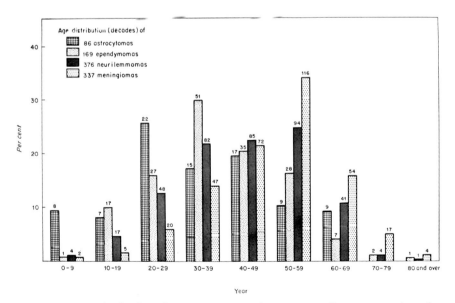

Figure 15. Distribution of astrocytomas, ependymomas, neurilemmomas and meningiomas on the basis of decades of age of patients.

Table 11. *Incidence of 86 Intramedullary Astrocytomas Based Upon Vertebral Level of Location*

Location	Grade				Total
	1	2	3	4	
Cervical	8	3	5	1	17
Cervicothoracic	7	3	–	1	11
Thoracic	23	12	4	2	41
Thoracolumbar	4	3	5	1	13
Lumbar	3	–	1	–	4

Location and Extent of the Lesions. Forty-one of the 86 astrocytomas were found in the thoracic area of the spinal column (Table 11); 11 others involved both the cervical and thoracic areas of the spinal column, and 13 others, the thoracic and lumbar areas. Only four were found in the lumbar area and 17 in the cervical area. It appears that this finding is in fairly close agreement with the expected incidence on the basis of the vertebral level (Table 4). Eighty per cent of the tumors were located in the combined cervical and thoracic areas; the expected incidence, on the basis of the vertebral level, would be 74 per cent. Sixty-seven per cent of the tumors were found in the combined thoracic and lumbar regions of the spinal column; this percentage would be expected to be 76. The occurrence of only four tumors in the lumbar area of the spinal column in our series is far less than would be expected, but this is not surprising. For instance, in Ravenel's calculations of the lesions which might be expected to arise in the lumbar portion of the spinal cord, he gave no consideration to the much smaller mass of the filum terminale in that vertebral level.

In the surgical cases the length of the tumor had to be estimated on the basis of the extent of the laminectomy, since often no other data were available in the records. Of course, the length of the laminectomy should not be considered as an accurate indication of the extent of the tumor itself. Most often the tumor will have been smaller than the length of the laminectomy, since the surgeon as a rule tries to extend the laminectomy to above and below the lesion which he sees. It appears that three-fourths of the astrocytomas required laminectomy which included four laminae or fewer. Three tumors extended over 10 or more vertebral levels. There was no indication that the more malignant neoplasms were larger or more extensive than those of a lower malignancy. In Figure 16 the location and extent of laminectomy as performed in all cases in which data were available have been given.

Preoperative Duration (Table 12). The preoperative duration of

Table 12. *Average Preoperative Duration of Symptoms and Average Postoperative Survival Periods Among 85 Patients Who Had Astrocytomas, Grades 1 to 4*

Grade	Spinal Cord Duration, Average				Filum Terminale Duration, Average				Total
	Preoperative		Postoperative		Preoperative		Postoperative		
	Cases	Months	Cases	Months	Cases	Months	Cases	Months	
1	42	39	35	101	2	108	1	276	
2	20	29	18	44	1	48	1	324	
3	12	7	9	16	3	8	2	15	
4	5	4	5	12	-	-	-	-	
Totals	79				6				85

symptoms among the 41 patients who had a grade 1 astrocytoma of the spinal cord was 39 months. In one patient, an astrocytoma grade 1 was found incidentally at necropsy. The similar period among those patients who had grade 2 astrocytomas was 29 months; among those who

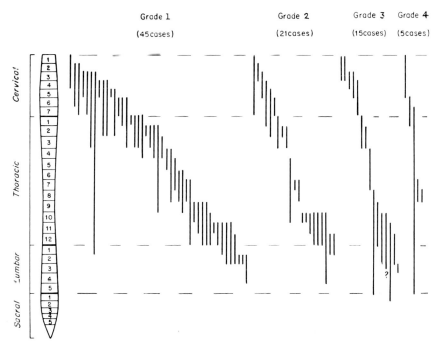

Figure 16. Anatomic location and extension of 86 astrocytomas of the spinal cord, grades 1 to 4.

had grade 3 astrocytomas it was 7 months; among those who had grade 4 astrocytomas it was only 4 months. It would thus appear that the time which elapsed between the first appearance of symptoms and the time operation was performed diminished as the malignancy of the lesions increased, an observation which applies also to astrocytomas of the brain. The variation in duration of symptoms among individual patients appeared to be wider when lesions were of lower malignancy than when they were of higher malignancy. Among patients who had grade 1 lesions this variation ranged from a month to 12 years, but in more than half the cases the time was 2 years or less. Among patients who had grade 2 lesions the shortest duration of symptoms was 2 months and the longest was 10 years, but in half of all the patients the preoperative duration of symptoms was a year or less. Seventy-five per cent of those who had grade 3 astrocytomas had experienced symptoms for less than a year; the longest time was 1½ years. The symptoms of four patients who had grade 4 astrocytomas existed for 5 months or less, and in only one other patient did this period reach 11 months. Details concerning the few cases in which the tumor was located in the filum terminale can be found in Table 12.

Postoperative Survival.   It would appear, on the basis of data in Table 12, that the postoperative survival period of patients who have astrocytomas is closely related to the grade of histologic malignancy. Among the 35 postoperative patients who had a grade 1 astrocytoma concerning whom subsequent details were known, the average length of survival was 101 months, and 24 patients, or approximately 68 per cent, died within this period. Among the 20 patients who had grade 2 lesions of the spinal cord the average length of survival of 18 was 44 months, and 14 patients (82 per cent) died within this period. Nine patients who had grade 3 astrocytomas of the spinal cord survived for an average of 16 months, and six of them (66 per cent) died before this time had elapsed. The length of survival of patients with grade 4 astrocytomas was even shorter, for, although the average length of survival was 12 months, four of five patients died within 7 months. One patient lived for 3 years after his first operation; however, he received two courses of extensive roentgen-ray treatment and finally had undergone cordectomy. The first surgical specimen examined in this case was of grade 3 malignancy, but at this time of cordectomy most of the tumor was of grade 4 malignancy.

The longest postoperative survival period among patients who had grade 1 astrocytomas was 31 years (our case 2), but it was unknown whether or not this patient was still alive at the time of this writing. Another 17 patients of the original 42 who were operated upon were reported to be alive at the time of this study; the average length of survival in this group was slightly more than 13 years. Only two patients of 21 who had grade 2 astrocytomas were known to be alive at the time of this study, and the longest survival time—17 years—was achieved by a patient with this grade of astrocytoma in the filum terminale; it had been thought that the lesion had been completely removed. Only one patient out of 15 who had grade 3 astrocytomas was known to be alive 2 years after operation. The longest survival in this group was achieved by a man who died 5 years after operation. No patient was alive among those who had had grade 4 astrocytomas and, as mentioned above, the longest period of survival in this group was 3 years.

We were interested in determining whether there was a relationship between the length of postoperative survival and the extent of the treatment. In Table 13 we grouped the patients on the basis of the type of operation performed and on the basis of whether or not roentgen-ray treatment was administered. The results of this comparison are very confusing and are inconclusive. This lack of clear-cut, significant results might be attributed partially to the small size of the subgroups, but it might also result because the final outcome of the tumor concerned is little influenced by the therapy.

Interpretation becomes even more complicated when the cause of death among patients who have tumors of the spinal cord is considered. It appears that the direct cause of death usually is a complication of the disease of the spinal cord. In the earlier cases in our series the renal problems often appeared to be of importance. They finally resulted in uremia. This complication is not so great a problem at present, but it still persists. Another complication, similarly more prominent in the past than now, was the development of trophic and decubital ulcers which can result in septicemia. A more direct relationship to the cause of death is progression of the symptoms, particularly the paralysis. Increase in paralysis may be caused by expansion or extension of the tumor, but it also can result from metastasis. Extension of the tumor should be more likely to cause a serious complication when it takes place in the vicinity of the vital centers, such as the cervical portion of the spinal cord. However, the data in Table 14, in which the survival time is charted against the vertebral levels of the lesions, do not support this concept.

In seven patients recurrence or progression, or both, of the symptoms necessitated reoperation.

Symptoms. Pain as the first symptom was present in 49 of the 85 cases. It was reported 23 times by patients who had grade 1 lesions, 16 times by those who had grade 2 lesions, nine times by those who had grade 3 tumors, and only once by a patient who had grade 4 astrocytomas. Twenty-five patients indicated that the pain was manifest in the back, nine reported it in the region of the neck, and seven said it occurred in one leg or both legs. Pain in the shoulder or arm was reported three times in each location. One patient complained of pain in the chest, and another reported headache.

Table 13. *Survival Time and Percentage of Survival of 63 Patients With Astrocytomas in Relation to Extent and Nature of Therapy*

Treatment, Type	\multicolumn{4}{Astrocytoma, Grade 1}													Total
			Alive				Alive				Alive				Alive	
	No.	Average Survival, Months	No.	Per Cent	No.	Average Survival, Months	No.	Per Cent	No.	Average Survival, Months	No.	Per Cent	No.	Average Survival, Months	No.	Per Cent	
Total removal	2	72	1	50	2	78	1	50	–	–	–	–	–	–	–	–	
Subtotal removal	3	44	3	100	5	33	1	20	3	4	0	0	–	–	–	–	
Biopsy	4	123	2	50	3	47	0	0	1	18	0	0	1	7	0	0	
Total removal and roentgen therapy	3	240	3	100	–	–	–	–	2	15	0	0	1	5	0	0	
Subtotal removal and roentgen therapy	10	79	4	40	3	12	1	33	2	43	0	0	1	7	0	0	
Biopsy and roentgen therapy	10	92	5	50	5	56	2	40	1	7	0	0	1	6	0	0	
Totals	32				18				9				4				63

The character of the pain was described variously as pain, aching, soreness, or discomfort.

Disturbance of motor function appeared as the first symptom in 25 cases. Such disturbance appeared as the first symptom in 14 patients who had a grade 1 lesion; in five who had a grade 2 tumor; in three who had a grade 3 neoplasm, and in three who had a grade 4 astrocytoma. In 21 patients motor dysfunction had developed in the legs; in the remaining four it had taken place in the hands or arms. The character of the disturbance was described variously as stiffness, spasticity, and difficulty in walking or in the use of the arms; sometimes it was reported as a tired or heavy feeling in the legs. One patient said that fibrillary twitchings were the first symptoms noted.

Nine patients said that sensory disturbance was the first symptom. This was reported as having occurred four times in the legs, three times in the arms, once in the neck, and once in the chest. Usually it was described as a sensation of numbness, tingling, or cold.

One patient said that the first sign noted was constipation, and another reported urinary incontinence as the initial manifestation.

The first time the patients were seen at the Mayo Clinic the symptoms were more extensive, and as a rule concurrent disturbance of several functions was detected. At the time of physical examination only three patients had pain as the only symptom, with the exception of some reflex changes. Fifty-six patients had pain which was associated with other disturbances; in 42 the disturbance included both motor and sensory

Table 14. *Survival Time, 70 Patients With Astrocytomas, Correlated With Location of Lesions in the Spinal Cord*

Location, Level of Spinal Column	Grade								Total
	1		2		3		4		
	No.	Survival, Months	No.	Survival, Months	No.	Survival, Months	No.	Survival, Months	
Cervical	5	115	2	80	4	9	1	7	
Cervico-thoracic	6	159	3	48	–	–	1	4	
Thoracic	19	86	10	25	3	18	2	7	
Thoraco-lumbar	4	132	3	79	4	25	1	36	
Lumbar	2	142	–	–	–	–	–	–	
Totals	36		18		11		5		70

Table 15.   *Average Protein Content of the Cerebrospinal Fluid Correlated With Degree of Obstruction of Fluid:*
60 Astrocytomas, Grades 1 to 4

Condition of Fluid	Grade								Totals	
	1		2		3		4			
	No.	Average Protein, mg., %	No.	Average Protein, mg., %	No.	Average Protein, mg., %	No.	Average Protein, mg., %	No.	Average Protein, mg., %
No block	20	503	7	325	7	607	-	-	34	487
Partial block	6	166	2	515	1	90	-	-	9	235
Total block	8	759	6	1935	2	1075	1	600	17	1202
Totals	34		15		10		1		60	

functions; in eight only sensory disturbance was involved and in six only motor dysfunction was demonstrated. Twenty-two patients had combined disturbances of the motor and sensory functions without pain; three patients were found to have only motor dysfunction, and in one disturbance of the sensorium was the only positive finding. Fourteen patients also were recorded as having incompetence of the sphincters of the bladder or bowel. Changes in tendon reflexes, either hyperreflexia or hyporeflexia, were found in 77 cases.

Cerebrospinal Fluid.   Spinal puncture had been done for 68 patients. In 21 instances complete block, and in nine instances incomplete block, of the cerebrospinal fluid was demonstrated. The average protein content of the cerebrospinal fluid in 60 cases was 652 mg. per 100 cc., and the average number of cells per cubic millimeter of fluid, recorded in 65 cases, was 7.

An analysis of the significance of partial block, total block, or no block of the cerebrospinal fluid in relation to the protein content (Table 15) indicates, as might be anticipated, that the protein content is greater when total block of the cerebrospinal fluid is present.

In only five patients of the total number who had astrocytomas was the protein content of the cerebrospinal fluid found to be within the normal range of 40 mg. per 100 cc. In 13 the protein content averaged between 40 and 100 mg. per 100 cc., and in 34 patients it was between 100 and 1000 mg. In eight it was more than 1000 mg. No striking differences could be detected between the content of protein in the cerebrospinal fluid in the several grades of astrocytomas.

Roentgenologic examination of the spinal column was done in 74 patients. In only five patients was this procedure diagnostic of tumor of the spinal cord, and in two instances it was doubtful.

Myelograms were made for 40 patients; results were negative in only one instance and were doubtful in another.

Scoliosis was found in 11 cases, and spina bifida, in two.

Papilledema was diagnosed in three patients: one had a grade 1 astrocytoma extending from the second to the sixth cervical vertebrae; one had a grade 1 astrocytoma extending from the seventh cervical to the first lumbar vertebrae; one had a grade 3 astrocytoma extending from the third to the fourth cervical vertebrae.

In 21 patients the surgeon noted the presence of a cyst in or adjacent to the tumor. It is interesting to find that 19 of these patients had a grade 1 astrocytoma and that only two had a grade 2 astrocytoma. In 10 instances histologic evidence indicated that the cyst probably was a part of a syringomyelic cavity. The relationship of tumors of the spinal cord to syringomyelia will be discussed in Chapter IV.

In our series we found three tumors which, in histologic structure, manifested outstanding features which distinguished them from ordinary astrocytomas. They appeared to be compatible with tumors of similar description in the literature, the subependymal glioma and the polar spongioblastoma. These two at present are recognized as specific entities, but there is no common opinion as to their origin or their place in the several classifications.

SUBEPENDYMAL GLIOMAS

This tumor is given different names in the literature. It was first recognized as an entity by Scheinker[251] in 1945. Under the name of "subependymoma" he described seven cases, in all of which the lesions were located in the brain.

Similar descriptions of this tumor form are to be found, however, in earlier literature, such as in Cox[56] in 1933 and in Riskaer[234] in 1944.

Under the title of "subependymal glomerate astrocytoma" Boykin and associates[24] (1954) reported nine cases, in two of which the lesions were located in the cervical portion of the spinal cord. According to these authors, this type of tumor is easily distinguished from other types of glioma because it is composed primarily of dense, interlacing bundles of neuroglia-like fibrils with clusters of nuclei, surrounded by ill-defined cytoplasm, scattered between these bundles.

There is no common opinion concerning the cell of origin of these neoplasms, although most investigators agree that they arise in the subependymal layer. The extremely rich matrix of fibrils suggests that the tumor is of astrocytic origin, but the nuclei, the structure, and the arrangement of the nuclei seem more to resemble those of ependymal cells. Boykin thought it most likely that these tumors are a variety of astrocytomas; this idea is partly supported by the study of McDonald[192] (1957).

Russell and Rubinstein[246] (1959) regarded these tumors as ependymomas in which the fibrillary subependymal astrocytes play an exceptionally active part, and they apparently were able, in contrast to Boykin and associates, to demonstrate the presence of blepharoplasts.

We found two examples of this type of tumor in our series. One was found incidentally at necropsy in a patient who also had a cellular ependymoma situated at a higher level in the cord and syringomyelia which involved nearly all of the cord. A more detailed description of this case is given in Chapter IV (case 21).

The other patient was a 48-year-old man who had noticed, 6 years before he was operated upon in 1957, impotence and a sensation of tightness around the abdomen. Later a sensory disturbance developed below the ribs, and weakness of both legs was reported. At examination it was found that reflexes in the legs were almost absent, and Babinski's sign was elicited bilaterally. The protein content of the cerebrospinal fluid was 500 mg. per 100 cc., and a myelogram disclosed complete block at the level of the first lumbar vertebra. A specimen of tissue was taken for biopsy. The surgeon noticed an intramedullary cyst situated above the tumor and extending as far as the eighth or ninth thoracic vertebra. The patient died at home $1\frac{1}{2}$ years after operation.

Histologic examination of the surgical specimen showed the tumor to be extremely rich in fibrils (staining as astroglia), with an occasional nucleus which resembled that of an astrocyte. In this fibrillar mass clumps of typical ependymal cells were found which sometimes had the characteristics of a rosette formation.

POLAR SPONGIOBLASTOMA

Russell and Rubinstein[246] (1959) discussed extensively the characteristics of a tumor group designated as "polar spongioblastoma" by Bailey and Cushing.[16] For several reasons Russell and Rubinstein regarded this tumor type as a variety of astrocytoma. On theoretic grounds they developed a new definition for what they called "true polar spongioblastomas"; that is, they wrote that this tumor "should be composed of tapering short and slender cells containing scanty and very fine neuroglial fibrils." The behavior of this tumor should be more aggressive, indicating its more primitive nature.

In earlier studies Russell and Cairns[245] (1947) and Russell[244] (1955) reported four such neoplasms as occurring in the brain.

We had one instance of this type of lesion in which most areas appeared to be similar to the tumors described by Russell. In some fields, however, the tumor showed all the characteristics of a low-grade astrocytoma. More details of this case are given in Chapter IV (case 18).

EPENDYMOMAS

Ependymal cells are those which are supposed to form the lining of the internal spaces of the central nervous system. The shape of the normal, non-neoplastic ependymal cell apparently is susceptible to variation, and it differs somewhat in the several locations of the nervous system. Normally, the thickness of the ependymal lining consists of only one cell layer, and the cellular form varies from a flattened to a cylindric appearance. Most commonly it is described as a polyhedral carrot-shaped cell with a moderate amount of cytoplasm and a nucleus that is located near the large end of the cell. According to Ranson and Clark[223] (1959), the ependymal cell has a fine, tail-like process which extends into the subependymal layer. In the adult person this process reaches the surface of the spinal cord only along the posterior median septum and in the anterior median fissure. This process does not stain with the ordinary neuroglial stains. During a period of development of the human embryo the free surface of the ependymal cell becomes ciliated, and at the base of each cilium a small granule is found which is known as a "blepharoplast." Blepharoplasts (sometimes several grouped together) are located under the surface of the cell, and they persist rather often, even though the cilia may have disappeared. The presence of blepharoplasts has been emphasized by Mallory[191] (1902) as a distinguishing feature of ependymomas. This view, however, was not accepted by Bailey[9] (1924), who also indicated that similar structures are found in the pineal and subependymal cells. The subject would seem to be a matter of considerable controversy, since Fletcher-Kernohan and one of us (Kernohan)[144] in 1937 observed that these granules were lacking in many ependymomas with ordinary staining methods, and since Russell and Rubinstein[246] (1959) wrote: "As a hallmark their [blepharoplasts] identification is of great importance, but often, it must be admitted, a matter of considerable difficulty."

The varying morphologic aspects of the normal ependymal cell also can be observed when the cells become dislocated, and no longer serve as lining cells of a normal cavity. In such an event they either form irregular clusters of dispersed polygonal cells or they become grouped around a small lumen. These patterns often are prominent in the occipital pole of the brain and in the area of the central canal of the spinal cord.

According to a study of Brown[33] (1939), obliteration of the central canal of the spinal cord is a fairly common process which starts shortly after birth and continues with the aging of the individual, so that by the age of 30 years, in 95 per cent of people, the central canal is obliterated. Brown suggested that obliteration is brought about by proliferation of the neuroglia of the substantia grisea. Although Brown wrote that no evidence was found that proliferation or metaplastic hyperplasia plays a role in the process of obliteration, his view was not accepted by Cornil and Mosinger[54] (1933). The difference of opinion might be the result of a varying interpretation of the changing morphologic aspects of the ependymal cell. Still, it cannot be denied that in certain cases in which the central canal is obliterated there appears to be an increase in the number of the ependymal cells. Accurate assessment is difficult, since even a patent central canal is also often surrounded by clusters of ependymal cells which do not constitute any part of the lining of a cavity. A different situation is encountered in the distal end of the spinal cord, beneath the point of emergence of the last two coccygeal nerves. At this site is found the ventriculus terminalis, a structure which is regarded as a true analogue of the ventricles of the brain. The walls, according to a study by one of us [Kernohan[140] (1924)], are irregular in outline, and around this ventriculus terminalis, as well as scattered in the filum terminale, many groups of ependymal cells are found, sometimes as solid clusters and sometimes forming small, canal-like structures.

So far as we know, the first description recognizable as that of an ependymoma, although the author's interpretation is different, is a report which Besold[20] made in 1896. Other similar descriptions of this period are those of Rosenthal[239] (1898) and of Storch[274] (1899). It was Mallory[191] in 1902 and Muthmann and Sauerbeck[199] in 1903 who recognized the relationship between certain types of gliomas and the ependymal cells. In the ensuing years many reports of cases were published, but in a critical analysis of all these reports Bailey[9] (1924) could identify only five lesions which were acceptable to him as true ependymomas. In 1925[10] he divided the tumors of this group into ependymomas and ependymoblastomas, but in 1927[11] he wrote that this distinction might be abandoned, from a clinical standpoint. He said, "All the tumors of this group are benign and cause trouble largely from their situation." It seemed to him that if any distinction should be made, it should be made on the basis of malignancy.

In 1931 Woltman, Adson, and one of us (Kernohan)[150] divided the ependymomas, on histologic and architectural grounds, into epithelial, myxopapillary, and cellular types. The term, "ependymoblastoma," in use by most neuropathologists, at this time was reserved to indicate the more malignant lesions.

In a study by Mabon, Svien, Craig, and one of us [Kernohan[185] (1949)], it was recognized that no correlation exists between the histologic classification in use until that time and the biologic behavior of these tumors in the brain. By analysis on the basis of anaplasia, it became evident that four grades of malignancy could be recognized. Since these four grades form the basis of the classification used in this study, we quote the descriptions as they were originally published in 1949.

Grade 1: . . . The tumor cells appear to be normal ependymocytes and the various architectural patterns such as the perivascular actiniform arrangement, the pseudorosette formation and the papillary patterns are well formed. There was no evidence of anaplasia as manifested by pleomorphism of the cytoplasm and nucleus hyperchromatism or the presence of mitotic figures.

Grade 2: . . . The architectural pattern is less distinct . . . but is readily discernible. The great majority of the component cells are normal-appearing ependymocytes. The remaining cells show evidence of early anaplastic transformation, as manifested by slight to moderate pleomorphism of the cytoplasm and nuclei, and hyperchromatism of the nuclei. No mitotic figures are present.

Grade 3: . . . The architectural pattern is still discernible but appears somewhat fragmentary. About one half of the component cells are normal-appearing ependymocytes. The remaining cells show evidence of moderate pleomorphism of the cytoplasm and nuclei, and hyperchromatism of the nuclei. Mitotic figures are present . . . at least one in every other high-power field.

Grade 4: . . . Only a small number of the cells are normal-appearing ependymocytes. The architectural patterns are presented only as remnants, and the tumor as a whole presents a disorganized picture. The remaining cells show evidence of marked pleomorphism of cytoplasm and nuclei, and hyperchromatism of the nuclei. Mitotic figures are abundant, averaging 4 or 5 per high-power field.

Gross Findings

Ependymomas of the spinal cord form an elongated-to-cylindric mass which is located inside and as a rule is completely surrounded by a sheet, variable in thickness, of more or less normal spinal-cord tissue. The cord appears to be swollen (Fig. 1) and often it fills the entire subarachnoid space. Occasionally the dura is stretched and thinned. When such changes are at hand the normal pulsations of the cerebrospinal fluid are not transmitted to levels below the level of the tumor, and the absence of these pulsations in the segment in question can be an important guide to the surgeon. Rather often the vessels situated below the site of the tumor are distended; occasionally they are somewhat tortuous. Sometimes the tumor breaks through the pia mater and extends into the subarachnoid space. If the tumor develops in the filum terminale it appears either as a fusiform swelling located somewhere along the course of that structure or as nodules attached to it (Fig. 17). The color of a fresh section of tumor is dependent upon the blood content; it varies from brownish-red to bluish-gray. Frequently there is a clear line of cleavage between the neoplasm and substance of the spinal cord, and sometimes the tumor is described as appearing to be encapsulated. The appearance of encapsulation is seen more often when the lesion arises in the filum terminale, but even in that situation, the tumor occasionally is seen to have ruptured through the original wall and to be growing diffusely between the roots of the cauda equina. Well-circumscribed tumors can be enucleated and removed totally, but the surgical treatment of those which are growing diffusely is difficult, hazardous, and often of necessity incomplete.

Generally, the consistency of the neoplasm is moderately soft and friable. Grossly the lesion has a granular, cauliflower-like appearance. The cut surface has the same granular, placenta-like structure. At times cysts are present in the neoplasm, but, surgically at least, they appear to

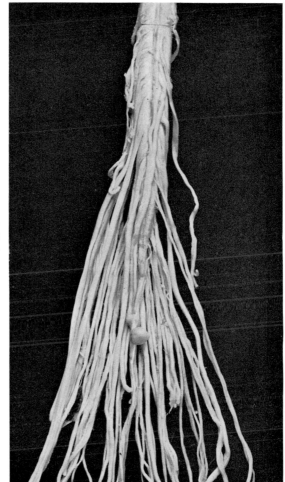

Figure 17. Two ependy-momas attached to the filum terminale in case 26 in Chapter IV.

be encountered more often at the borders, chiefly at the upper and lower poles of the tumor. In a number of cases we have histologic proof that these cysts are not tumor-cysts but are syringomyelic cavities. The relationship of these structures to the tumors will be discussed in more detail in Chapter IV.

Hemorrhage and softening of the tissue sometimes are found, even in tumors of a low-grade malignancy. It is possible for calcification to develop, but it can be considered to be rare in the gross specimen.

Histologic Aspects

Grade 1 Ependymoma, Cellular Type. The cellular ependymoma is the most common type of all ependymomas of the spinal cord and filum terminale, taken together. It is absolutely the most frequent of all types of ependymomas occurring in the spinal cord; it occurs almost as frequently as the papillary type in the filum terminale. Many ependymo-mas are of a mixed type, and it is not uncommon to find in a cellular ependymoma areas which are representative of the papillary or epithelial type.

The main structure of the cellular ependymoma is a mosaic-like pat-tern which suggests a crowding-together of a polygonal type of cell. The nuclei are distinctly larger than those of astrocytes; they are rather plump and possess a clear nuclear membrane. The nuclei vary slightly between oval and round; sometimes they may be slightly elongated. No pleomorphism of any significance is seen. The nuclei have a mod-erate content of chromatin which is, as a rule, condensed into moder-ately coarse, irregular granules scattered in the karyoplasm. Sometimes the chromatin appears to be collected chiefly beneath the nuclear mem-brane, giving the nucleus a vesicular appearance. Nucleoli, several of which at times are seen in one nucleus, often can be recognized, but visualization of the nucleoli seems to be influenced by the staining method which is employed. The presence of nuclear vacuoles is not un-common; in rare instances purple-reddish homogeneous so-called inclu-sion bodies can be detected.

Generally, the nuclei are surrounded by abundant cytoplasm which often has a coarse, granular or a smooth, eosinophilic appearance, but which sometimes is vacuolated. These vacuoles do not stain specifically for mucus or glycogen, although we found that occasionally the muci-carmine stain gave a faint pink reaction, which was not, however, strong enough to be considered a positive reaction. Cellular outlines, espe-

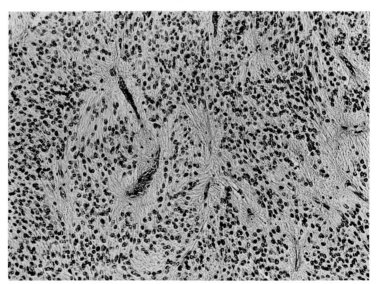

Figure 18. A grade 1 ependymoma of the cellular type. Uniform cell masses are interrupted by clear perivascular spaces composed of fibrils (hem-atoxylin and eosin; × 125).

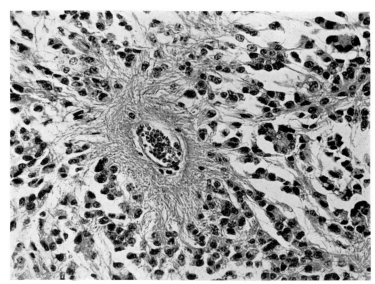

Figure 19. A grade 1 ependymoma of the cellular type. There is a nuclear-free cuff around a blood vessel; at the right is a small rosette (hematoxylin and eosin; × 300).

cially in the densely packed tumors, as a rule are either absent or can be discerned only vaguely; once in a while, however, clear cellular membranes can be seen, and the mosaic pattern becomes more apparent. No cellular processes are found in these areas. The uniform monotonous pattern is interrupted by vessels (Fig. 18). It is here that the most characteristic pattern of the cellular ependymoma is found: it consists of a perivascular arrangement of the tumor cells. The ependymal cells are radially oriented around the blood vessels (Fig. 19) and all the nuclei remain at a certain distance from the vessel. The zone immediately around the blood vessel does not contain nuclei; thus the typical arrangement of a nuclei-free cuff around the vessel is produced which is easily recognized in these fairly cellular tumors. The nuclei-free zone is composed solely of tail-like cellular processes of slightly variable thickness and density. These processes appear to be attached to the vascular adventitia, however, without having a well-formed vascular foot. One cell rarely has more than one process, and the processes seldom branch. The processes do not contain neuroglial fibrils. This can be demonstrated with the Mallory phosphotungstic acid hematoxylin stain, and they do not become impregnated when they are subjected to Cajal's gold chloride method.

Incidentally, other diagnostic patterns can be encountered in a cellular ependymoma. One of these is the rosette formation (Fig. 20), in which several ependymal cells are arranged around a small open space which occasionally contains some protein-rich fluid. Most often these cells

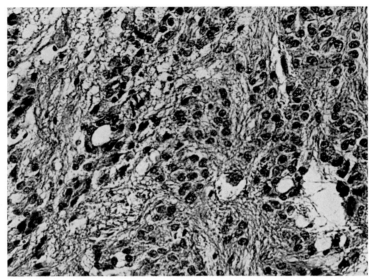

Figure 20. A grade 1 ependymoma of the cellular type, with rosettes (hematoxylin and eosin; × 350).

display clear cellular membranes; the cellular form is mostly cuboidal or cylindric. Another pattern which can be present is the pseudorosette formation in which the ependymal cells are arranged radially around a center without an open space. In such an instance these cells appear more as an elongated type, without distinct cellular borders.

The compact cell masses sometimes are separated by wavering bands of thin, crisscrossing fibers (Fig. 21) which convey the impression of felt-work which varies in compactness. These bands contain few nuclei. Usually it is not possible to demonstrate that these bands are glial fibrils, since, except for an occasional fiber, they do not react to the ordinary neuroglial stains. The number of these structures is extremely variable in the various tumors, and this variation also holds true in respect to different areas in the same tumor. Interesting structures often, but not always, related to these masses of fibers are small, fairly round, eosin-staining bodies (Fig. 22). These bodies, commonly referred to as "balloons," do not show any relationship to cells; they are not sharply circumscribed, and they have borders which often appear to be prickly. The centers of these bodies sometimes stain with a weaker intensity than do the borders, but there are no laminations. They do not have a specific affinity for silver; they stain pink with the Mallory phosphotungstic acid hematoxylin, and blue with the Mallory-Heidenhain stain. They give a weakly positive reaction to the mucin stain and are purple when treated with PAS stain (Fig. 23). The significance of these bodies is unknown, but they are found in varying numbers in some of the cellular ependy-

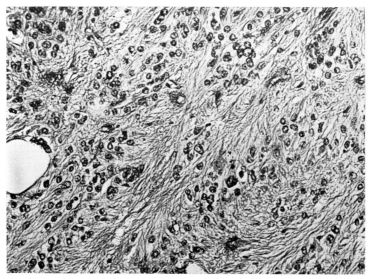

Figure 21. A grade 1 ependymoma of the cellular type, showing bands of crisscrossing fibrils separating the cellular areas (hematoxylin and eosin; × 175).

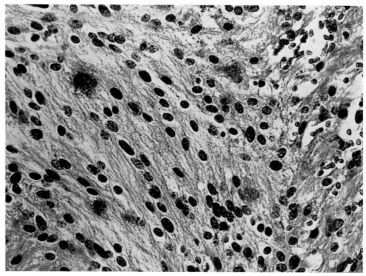

Figure 22. A grade 1 ependymoma of the cellular type, showing so-called balloons (hematoxylin and eosin; × 350).

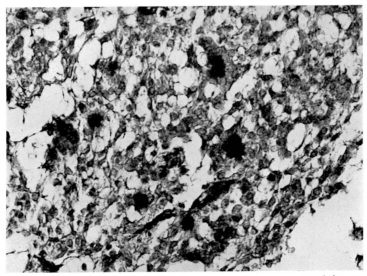

Figure 23. A grade 1 ependymoma of the cellular type, containing so-called balloons (PAS; × 350).

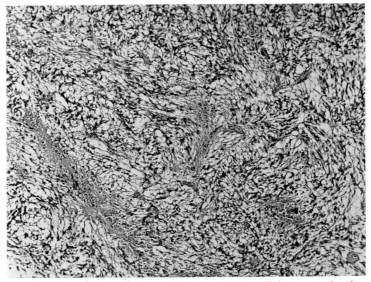

Figure 24. A grade 1 ependymoma of the cellular type, showing marked intercellular edema (hematoxylin and eosin; × 100).

momas but occasionally also in the papillary and epithelial types of ependymomas.

The architecture of the cellular ependymoma does not always have the pattern described above. Most of the additional variations can be related to a loosening of the compactness of the cellular structure (Fig. 24). A gradual change can be visualized in a series of tumors. Individual tumor cells become easier to recognize as a result of the cells having become separated from each other by intercellular spaces of varying size. The size of the intercellular spaces can be considerable, and can produce a histologic picture in which the ependymal cells become stretched out and almost form a reticular-like network with large, open meshes. These spaces, for the most part, are optically clear, but in an occasional one a faint, fine, granular eosinophilic structure can be visualized. We were unable to demonstrate any content, and we judge that the spaces are filled with a serous fluid or fluid like that seen when edema is present.

This process of "edematization" appeared to be more common and more extensive in tumors of the filum terminale than in tumors of the spinal cord.

By virtue of this process, delineation of the individual cells becomes easier, and several cell forms become apparent. There are cells of a polygonal form without cellular processes, but others are more elongated and are carrot-shaped, with one clear, fairly plump tail-like process, not unlike those seen in the perivascular spaces. There are also spindle-shaped cells which have a nucleus located in the thickest part of the middle of the cell. We were unable to demonstrate intracellular fibrils.

These highly edematous tumors can cause considerable differential diagnostic problems. In all instances, however, we were able to find additional structures, such as a perivascular arrangement (Fig. 25) or rosette formation (Fig. 26) to support the diagnosis of cellular ependymoma.

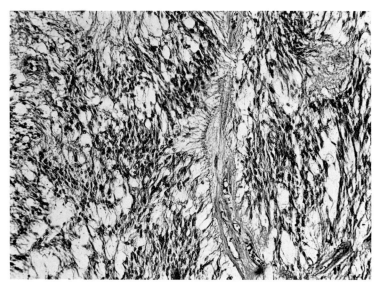

Figure 25. A grade 1 ependymoma of the cellular type, showing a perivascular structure in an edematous tumor (hematoxylin and eosin; × 125).

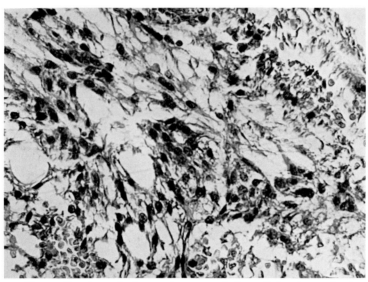

Figure 26. A grade 1 ependymoma of the cellular type, showing rosette formation in an edematous lesion (hematoxylin and eosin; × 400).

Another less common pattern consists of a fascicular, bundle-like arrangement of more elongated cells (Fig. 27). These bundles are interwoven. Sometimes they exhibit vague whorl formations. Occasionally there may even be a faint suggestion of palisading, so that the observer may be reminded of a neurilemmoma. Aids in differential diagnosis also are represented by the presence of perivascular structures or canal formation. Additional factors are that the nuclei are larger and more plump than those of neurilemmomas, and that Anthoni B-like tissue is absent.

Of undecided significance was the presence of cells which exhibited a completely clear or almost completely clear space between the nucleus and the apparent border of the cell. Some of these cells were found alone, but sometimes they were seen in groups, and in the latter instance the area had a honeycomb appearance such as is usually associated with oligodendrogliomas. The cytoplasm of these cells either did not stain at all or did so very faintly when treated with eosin or other stains. The nuclei of these cells tended to be smaller and more compact than ependymal nuclei, and the chromatin was slightly less granular and more evenly distributed through the nucleus. The presence of these cells may constitute a diagnostic problem, since we studied several tumors in which they were present in such abundance that we felt justified in making the diagnosis of "mixed glioma," "ependymoma with oligodendroglioma," or the reverse, depending on the cell type which was most dominant.

These oligodendroglia-like cells should not be confused with foam or

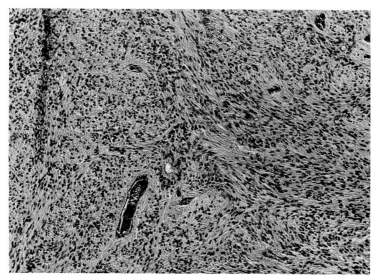

Figure 27. A grade 1 ependymoma of the cellular type. Note the fascicular, bundle-like arrangement of the ependymal cells with a perivascular arrangement and a rosette (hematoxylin and eosin; × 100).

xanthoma cells, which occasionally are present. Xanthoma cells have a smaller nucleus which is more condensed, and a diffuse, finely granular cytoplasm. We consider them to be phagocytic cells.

Another phenomenon of phagocytic activity is found in cells which contain a coarse, brown, granular pigment which gives a positive reaction to staining for iron. These cells are present fairly frequently. We believe they are the results of former smaller or larger hemorrhages.

The stroma of cellular ependymomas consists largely of vascular structures with little other connective tissue. Usually, the vessels are abundant; they vary considerably in size. Rather often the wall is thickened and is homogeneously pink; in this hyaline wall no nuclei are found. Even in the low-grade and slowly growing ependymomas there is sometimes a moderate increase in number and swelling of the endothelial cells of the blood vessels (Fig. 28). Rarely, several small vessels were seen which were surrounded by one hyaline membrane; the structure resembled slightly the glomerular-like structures of highly malignant astrocytomas.

Sometimes thrombosis in one or more vessels is seen, and the necrosis which we noted in several tumors probably was the result of this change.

Sometime calcification also is found; but if it is, as a rule it is slight, consisting of small granules in the stroma but seldom in the parenchyma of the tumors.

Grade 1 Ependymoma, Papillary Type. The papillary ependymoma is second in frequency of occurrence. Most examples of this type were located in the filum terminale; only a few had developed in the spinal

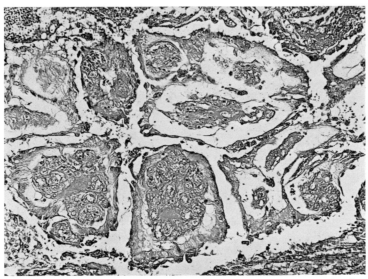

Figure 28. A grade 1 ependymoma of the papillary type, showing marked vascular and endothelial proliferation in a low-grade tumor (hematoxylin and eosin; × 150).

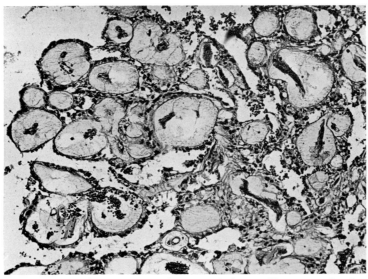

Figure 29. A grade 1 ependymoma of the papillary type, showing villi-like structure composed of a myxomatous, degenerated stroma with a centrally located vessel and covered by ependymal cells (hematoxylin and eosin; × 150).

cord. The common histologic architecture can be described as that of villi, which are composed of a central core of connective tissue and blood vessels surrounded mostly by a single layer of ependymal cells (Fig. 29). The nuclei of these ependymal cells are fairly large and are more commonly oval than round. The nuclear membrane is distinct. There is little or no pleomorphism, and there are no mitotic figures. The chromatin content of the nuclei sometimes appears to be slightly higher than in the cellular type, but it still can be considered moderate. The chromatin appears as fine, distinct granules, and rather often it is somewhat less coarse than in the cellular type of ependymomas. The chromatin granules are evenly distributed through the nucleus. Vesicular nuclei are seen in lesser numbers than in the cellular types. Nucleoli most often can be easily detected, although in our series they varied in frequency in the several tumors. Nuclear vacuoles occasionally are seen, but inclusion bodies are rare.

The form of the cells showed considerable variations (Fig. 30). In some places the cells appeared to be almost flattened, but in other areas cuboidal or cylindric forms were present. It was even not unusual to find cells with tail-like processes that were directed toward the center of the connective-tissue core. These processes varied greatly in length, but usually were short and heavy.

The amount of cytoplasm present varied according to the cellular form. Often it had a fine, granular appearance. Vacuoles occasionally were present; only very few of them reacted with a purple color to the

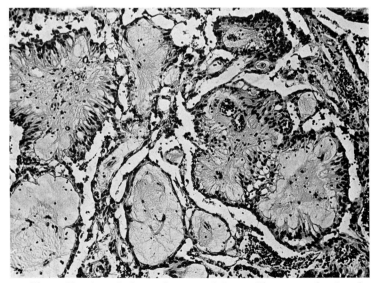

Figure 30. A grade 1 ependymoma of the papillary type, showing the varying sizes and shapes of the cells covering the villi (hematoxylin and eosin; × 100).

PAS stain and a pinkish-red reaction to the mucicarmine stain. The cellular borders were not always clearly indicated.

The ependymal cells surrounded a core of connective tissue, and sometimes they appeared to be separated from this by a pseudobasement membrane. A real basement membrane could not be demonstrated; this pseudobasement membrane had the staining characteristics of connective tissue.

The inner area of the villi consisted of connective tissue with a blood vessel in the center, although this latter was not a constant feature. The connective-tissue stroma often showed various stages of myxomatous degeneration. It was not uncommon even to find a complete disappearance of connective-tissue stroma and blood vessels, so that only a myxomatous material remained. This myxomatous material stained faint blue, purple, or pink with hematoxylin and eosin and stained specifically for mucus. The mucus is regarded as being the result of myxomatous degeneration of the connective tissue; it is separated from the ependymal cells by the pseudomembrane of connective tissue.

The form and the size of the villi exhibit considerable variation; they range from small round to large branched structures. Sometimes the villi are separated, resembling the placenta structure, but at other times they are interconnected. The smaller villi, although appearing to be independent when examined in a histologic section, are branches of larger structures, and the ultimate gross picture is papillary.

The architecture as described above is only one of the variations which

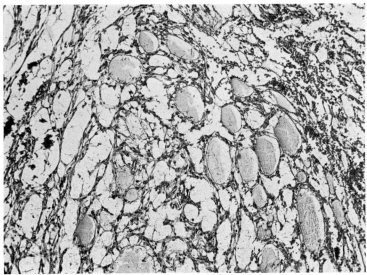

Figure 31. A grade 1 ependymoma of the papillary type. The structure is alveolar-like, and within the lumina is a bluish-pink material which stains positive for mucin (hematoxylin and eosin; × 100).

constitute papillary ependymomas. Another variation which is fairly common can be described best as "alveolar-like." It consists of a mesh-work of interconnected bundles of flattened ependymal cells (Fig. 31). The lumina they enclose usually are filled with a bluish-pink material which is seen to contain mucus after treatment with specific stains. The nuclear structures remain the same as in the first variation, but the cellular forms appear to be elongated. Sometimes the cells are flattened or cuboidal, and have an epithelial-like arrangement around the lumen. This formation sometimes can resemble the edematous structure of a cellular ependymoma. A characteristic difference, however, is that the open spaces in the papillary variant contain a mucinous material, slightly purple or bluish in hematoxylin and eosin stain and pink in mucicarmine stain. In addition, other papillary structures almost always can be found in different areas of the same tumor.

Another variation consists of an arborescent connective-tissue structure which is lined on all sides by one layer, or occasionally by several layers, of ependymal cells (Fig. 32). The essential cellular forms appear to be polygonal, with a short plump process which is directed toward the con-nective tissue. The cytoplasm is fairly abundant; usually it appears to be finely granular. The nucleus is located in the upper two-thirds portion of the cell; it varies from round to oval. The chromatin is finely granular and is evenly distributed over the nucleus. The cellular membranes often are not well demarcated. The cell layers covering adjacent connec-tive-tissue branches are not always separated by a clear, open space which divides them into two groups, each belonging to one connective-tissue

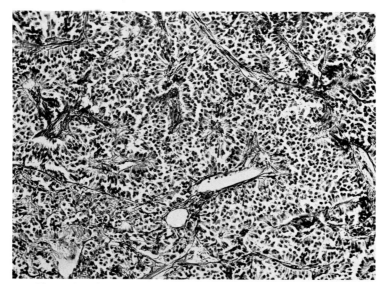

Figure 32. A grade 1 ependymoma of the papillary type, showing branching connective-tissue cores covered by ependymal cells (hematoxylin and eosin; × 150).

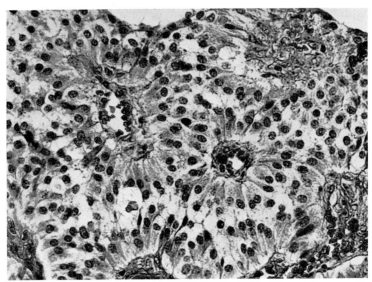

Figure 33. A grade 1 ependymoma of the papillary type. The centrally located blood vessels are surrounded by ependymal cells. Note the line of cleavage between the papillae and the cellular and nuclear structures (hematoxylin and eosin; × 350).

core, but fairly often a line of cleavage can be visualized which (Fig. 33) indicates the papillary nature of the tumor. In this particular variation of papillary ependymoma only rarely is there evidence of myxomatous degeneration of the connective tissue, and mucus is absent. The connective tissue contains a large number of small blood vessels, many of which are capillaries. There is seldom swelling or proliferation of the endothelial cells, but hyaline thickening of the vascular wall is not uncommon. When Mallory phosphotungstic acid stain or Holzer stain was used no evidence of neuroglial fibrils could be found.

In all the described variations of papillary ependymomas cellular patterns can be found which are more or less typical of the cellular ependymoma, and a perivascular arrangement also is found occasionally. Rosette formations, however, are extremely rare in this type of lesion.

Sometimes calcification is present; it involves mostly the walls of the blood vessels and rarely the parenchyma. Evidence of old hemorrhages is found in the presence of cells loaded with brown, granular, iron-positive pigment.

Grade 1 Ependymoma, Epithelial Type. The epithelial type of ependymoma is the easiest to recognize because some of the tumor cells are arranged in canals. In our series, however, this type of ependymoma was the least common of all ependymomas.

Typical structures of the epithelial ependymoma are numerous round or irregular-shaped cavities lined by cuboidal or columnar cells (Fig. 34). The size of these canals or cavities varies greatly, as does also the shape.

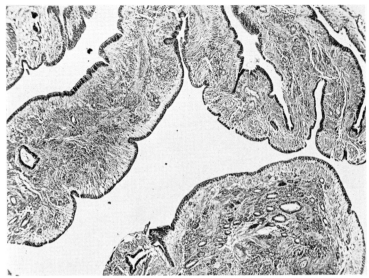

Figure 34. A grade 1 ependymoma of the epithelial type. Large, ir-regularly shaped clefts are lined by cuboidal or columnar ependymal cells (hematoxylin and eosin; × 30).

In the histologic sections the lumina of these cavities as a rule are opti-cally clear, but occasionally a pink, slightly granular or hyaline-like material is found. This material does not stain specifically for mucus. It probably represents a protein-containing fluid with some cellular debris. The small, round canals (Fig. 35) are identical to the rosettes found in the cellular ependymoma; they represent the tendency of the ependymal cells to line a cavity.

The nuclei of the lining cells are fairly large; their form varies be-tween oval and round. As a rule the chromatin appears to be finely granular, and is fairly evenly distributed over the karyoplasm. There is a distinct nuclear membrane. Vesicular nuclei seem to be rare, but nuclear vacuoles occasionally are seen. Nucleoli are present, but are not constant features. Mitosis is absent.

The form of the cells lining the cavities varies between cuboidal and high columnar. Most often the nucleus is located at the opposite end of the free border of the cell. Sometimes the cellular outlines are easily recognized, but often they are indistinct, except where they touch the cavity. The cytoplasm appears as fine, regularly distributed granules. Cellular vacuoles are uncommon; when they do occur it is rare they will stain positively for mucus.

A number of the epithelial cells have a cellular process at the end opposite the cavity. These processes are fairly thick; they disappear mostly in the subepithelial tissue. At times some processes are directed toward an adjacent blood vessel, and they apparently end at the peri-

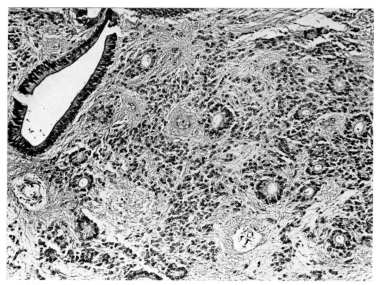

Figure 35. A grade 1 ependymoma of the epithelial type. Many rosettes and one larger space lined by epithelial-like ependymal cells are seen
(hematoxylin and eosin; × 100).

vascular space. Generally, a cell has only one process which does not
divide. In our series the Mallory phosphotungstic acid stain or the
Holzer stain did not demonstrate neuroglial fibrils. Occasionally the
epithelial cell appears to rest on a membrane-like structure, but we were
unable to confirm the presence of a basal membrane. There is also no
basal membrane or basal membrane-like structure between the free ends
of the cells and the lumina of the cavities or rosettes. An occasional cell
possesses cilia on its free surface; this feature, however, is an exception.
Blepharoplasts are seen fairly often in the lining cells of the cavities.

It is unusual to encounter a tumor in which all the ependymal cells
are arranged in this characteristic pattern. Usually, the tissue between
the cavities is composed of ependymal cells which are compressed into
irregular cell groups, and these cell groups are separated from each
other by blood vessels. Around the blood vessels the cells are arranged
radially, with a characteristic nuclear free zone. This pattern is identical
with that of the cellular ependymomas.

Although an abundance of blood vessels can be present, the amount of
connective tissue is minimal and is restricted to the walls of the vessels.
Sometimes the vascular walls are hyalinized, but endothelial swelling or
proliferation is rare.

In our series calcification was not found.

Grade 2 Ependymoma.   About a third of the ependymomas in our
series exhibited histologic features interpreted as being characteristic
of a higher degree of malignancy. This increased malignancy was mani-

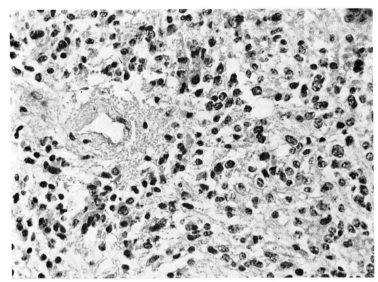

Figure 36. A grade 2 ependymoma of the cellular type. Increased pleomorphism and some degree of hyperchromatism indicate increased malignancy (hematoxylin and eosin; × 350),

fested mainly by anaplastic changes in a number of nuclei and cells. Most of the tumor cells, however, appeared to be more or less normal ependymal cells. The changes in the more malignant cells often were of minimal degree; they consisted mainly of slight-to-moderate pleomorphism of the nucleus (Fig. 36). Not only was there a more pronounced variation in the size of the nuclei, but the usual round-to-oval form was seen to have become slightly irregular. The nuclear membrane remained clearly indicated. The nuclear chromatin became either more coarsely granular (the granules being irregular in size and shape and darker in staining intensity) or appeared to be finer but more condensed, giving the nucleus a hyperchromatic aspect. Since only a small number of the nuclei showed these changes, the hyperchromatic ones stood out more clearly in histologic preparations. The nucleoli were difficult to visualize. As a rule, there were no mitotic figures.

In some cases there was a slight increase in the number of nuclei, but this was not always so. The decision as to cellularity can be difficult, since all ependymomas appear to be generally fairly cellular.

The same architectural patterns described for grade 1 ependymomas appear in grade 2 ependymomas, but the cellular arrangement appears relatively more frequently than in lesions of grade 1 malignancy. The cellular types sometimes appear to be more cellular (Fig. 37), and when the individual cells can be visualized it becomes apparent that there is also more variation in the size and shape of the cells and that the cytoplasm often is less abundant. Generally, there are fewer vacuoles

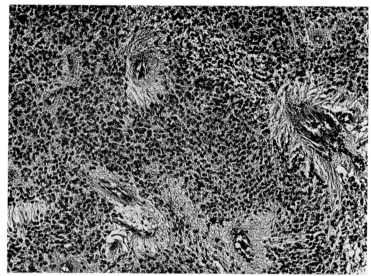

Figure 37. A grade 2 ependymoma of the cellular type. Slightly increased cellularity is seen with some degree of pleomorphism and hyperchromatism. The perivascular arrangement is preserved (hematoxylin and eosin; × 125).

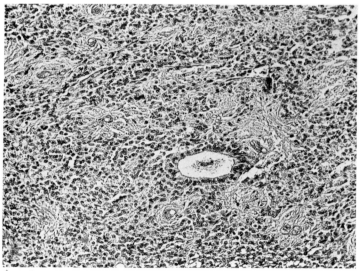

Figure 38. A grade 2 ependymoma of the cellular type, showing rosette formation (hematoxylin and eosin; × 150).

in the cells, but the cytoplasm appears to be finely granular. Intercellular vacuolization also is less prominent, and the tumors seldom show the loose arrangement which is a feature of grade 1 ependymomas. The rosette formation (Fig. 38) and pseudorosette formation occasionally are present, but they do not occur as regular features. The strands of crisscrossing fibrils and the so-called balloons previously described as features of grade 1 lesions also are less common. It might appear that these tumors are less well vascularized, but this impression results partially because the vessels do not stand out clearly, the perivascular arrangement (Fig. 39) being not so regular and pronounced. In general, the architectural patterns are less distinct but are still sufficiently recognizable.

In our series there were only a few grade 2 papillary ependymomas (Fig. 40). Cellular and nuclear pleomorphism was more marked in such lesions, but myxomatous degeneration of the connective stroma, although present, appeared to be less apparent and less extensive.

We had no lesion in our series which would fulfill the criteria of an epithelial ependymoma, grade 2, but several tumors exhibited smaller or larger irregular cavities lined by cells which displayed slight pleomorphism of cell and nucleus (Fig. 41) The cellular areas were, however, dominating, and anaplastic changes also were present in these areas.

Vascular changes are difficult to interpret, since endothelial swelling and proliferation sometimes are present, even in grade 1 ependymomas.

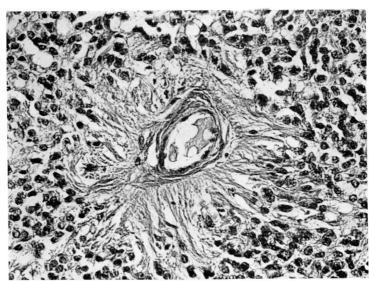

Figure 39. A grade 2 ependymoma of the cellular type. The perivascular arrangement persists, but there are also increased cellularity, pleomorphism and some degree of hyperchromatism (hematoxylin and eosin; × 350).

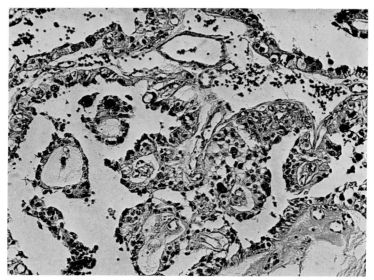

Figure 40.   A grade 2 ependymoma of the papillary type. Pleomorphism and hyperchromatism are increased (hematoxylin and eosin; × 150).

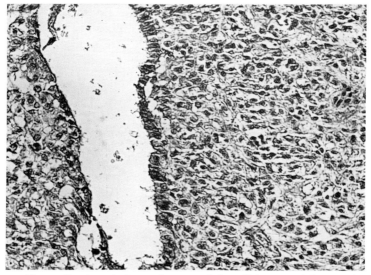

Figure 41.   A grade 2 ependymoma of the cellular type. A large cavity is lined by epithelial-like ependymal cells (hematoxylin and eosin; × 175).

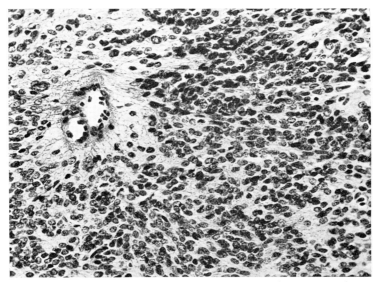

Figure 42. A grade 3 ependymoma of the cellular type. Moderate pleomorphism, slight hyperchromatism and several mitotic processes are seen. The perivascular arrangement is still preserved (hematoxylin and eosin; × 225).

It would appear, however, that these vascular changes are more prominent and that they increase as malignancy increases.

Grade 3 Ependymoma. It will perhaps be agreed that the placing of a gradual series of changes in cell and nucleus into four groups is somewhat unrealistic, and that it can cause indecision as to the final diagnosis, since it requires consideration of so many criteria. In our series there were only five examples of grade 3 ependymomas, and all appeared to be different. We did notice, however, a general tendency toward an increase in anaplastic changes in nuclei and cells (Fig. 42). In addition to marked variation in the sizes and shapes of fewer than half of all the nuclei, there was marked variation in the appearance of the chromatin. Sometimes it had the appearance of small, dustlike granules scattered irregularly throughout the nucleus, but usually we noticed an increase in the size of the granules, which formed dense aggregates which imparted the appearance of hyperchromatism to the nucleus. This change was more prominent in lesions of this grade than it was in grade 2 ependymomas. The nuclear membrane remained sharply outlined, but nucleoli became much more difficult to visualize. Mitosis was present in all the tumors, but the number of mitotic figures was variable. It is not unusual to find several multinucleated cells, and once in a while a giant nucleus is detected.

Cellularity appears to be moderately increased, and the cells are more closely packed together. In this grade of lesion the cytoplasm often is still finely granular, but vacuolization is uncommon. The cellular membranes seldom are clearly indicated. The cellular form appears to be variable, but the less anaplastic cells displayed normal shapes, such as were seen in tumors of less malignancy; that is, polygonal, carrot-shaped, or spindle-shaped.

The architectural patterns are still discernible (Fig. 43), but are becoming more fragmentary. These patterns can be extremely helpful in the diagnosis, and it is worth while to search for them. Best preserved are the indications of the perivascular arrangement, but they are less frequent and less well organized. In one of our six examples a pure papillary formation was seen, without myxomatous degeneration of the connective-tissue stroma; marked pleomorphism and hyperchromatism also were evident. In another lesion some irregular-shaped cavities lined with epithelial-like cells were seen, with, however, a marked anaplastic change of the cell and nucleus. The cellular areas in this tumor were dominant and highly cellular, with marked anaplasia and a fair number of mitotic figures.

It has already been emphasized that vascular changes in ependymomas constitute an unreliable guide to the degree of malignancy. Even in grade 3 ependymomas we found fairly normal vasculature, although hyalinized vessels were encountered, as were swelling and proliferation of the endothelial cells of the vessels.

Grade 4 Ependymoma.   We had no example of this type of tumor in our series.

Before entering into a detailed analysis of the data of our series, we

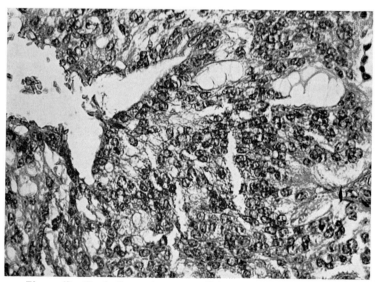

Figure 43.   Grade 3 ependymoma, cellular type. Despite the increased malignancy, there is an indication of a perivascular arrangement (right) and a cavity lined with ependymal cells (left) (hematoxylin and eosin; × 350).

shall present several reports of cases to show some of the peculiarities of the symptoms produced by these tumors. The first two cases concern grade 1 ependymomas, and the next two have to do with grade 2 ependymomas.

Report of Cases of Ependymomas

Case 6

A farmer 35 years old came to the Mayo Clinic in 1950; he gave a 3-year history that had started with the sudden onset of severe stiff neck. Movements of his head were restricted because of pain in the area of the neck. This episode lasted for about a month, and then gradually disappeared within 2 or 3 months. Eight months later he became aware of numbness in the right leg and trunk, and he also experienced dysphagia and nasal regurgitation. Again there was a period of improvement, but he never obtained complete relief from the subjective numbness. Shortly afterward he noted a low, substernal, sharp, knife-like pain when he was riding on farm machinery, and he experienced flashes of pain with each jolt. This pain also was induced by coughing or flexion of the neck. During the winter months the pain gradually ceased, but it returned during the next summer and again in the spring a year later. In addition, at this time he noted the onset of numbness in the left foot and a sensation such as might be imparted by a "tight elastic cloth" wrapped around his waist. Potentia coeundi was reduced; control of the bowel was poor, and the urinary stream was slow starting during the last few weeks before the patient was seen at the Mayo Clinic. His local physician carried out lumbar puncture and found the initial pressure of the cerebrospinal fluid to be 21 cm. of water with a slow increase to 35 cm. of water under jugular compression, but no decrease after release of the compression. The protein content of the cerebrospinal fluid, as determined by the local physician, was 115 mg. per 100 cc. The patient was referred to the Mayo Clinic with the diagnosis of tumor of the spinal cord.

Physical examination disclosed a varying degree of anesthesia below the nipple line, with total anesthesia over the lower part of the thorax and the abdomen and on the inner aspects of the upper third portions of the thighs. There was also a varying degree of analgesia and thermo-anesthesia in the same areas. Vibratory sense was diminished in the legs. Motor functions were essentially undisturbed. The abdominal reflexes were normal; symmetric hyperreflexia was elicited in the legs. The gait was slightly ataxic.

Myelography was done. Cephalad flow of the contrast medium was seen to be completely obstructed opposite the level of the inferior border of the third thoracic vertebra; the free margin of the defect was so irregular that the radiologist was unable to determine whether the tumor was intramedullary or extramedullary. It was also noted in the roentgenogram that the vessels at the site of the lesion were tortuous and increased in size. A vascular origin of the lesion was thought to be possible.

Laminectomy was then performed in which the spines and laminae of the second, third, and fourth thoracic vertebrae were removed. An extradural mass was not detected, but after the dura had been opened an intramedullary tumor was found. After the posterior columns had been split, a reddish, fairly encapsulated tumor, filling the central part of the cord from the first to the fourth thoracic vertebrae, was encountered and was removed as far as it could be detected grossly. The cord had been badly compressed by the lesion and had been replaced by the tumor for three-fourths of the width of the cord. Histologically, the tumor was diagnosed as a grade 1 ependymoma of the epithelial type.

The postoperative period was uneventful except that the patient had a minor cold.

Re-examination after 3 months showed marked improvement. Only slight spasticity of the right leg was noted, and a small area of diminished sensation to touch, and pain in the thorax, were demonstrated. At this time a course of roentgen-ray irradiation was given.

Ten years after the operation the patient's local physician reported that the patient had only minor residual neurologic changes in the form of slightly increased reflexes.

Case 7

A 12-year-old boy was first seen at the Mayo Clinic in 1949. At that time he complained chiefly of pain and stiffness, of a year's duration, in both legs. Half a year previously he had begun to experience pain in the eyes, blurred vision, and bilateral frontal headache. His local physician had noted, 2 weeks before the patient came here, bilateral papilledema and xanthochromic cerebrospinal fluid which clotted on standing.

The boy was found to be obese, but well developed. Neurologic examination revealed slight hyperreflexia in the right leg, bilateral spasm of the hamstring muscles, and contraction or spasm of the left knee. Examination of the eyes disclosed grade 4 papilledema, and large white exudates and hemorrhages were seen in both optic disks. The vision, pupils, and visual fields were normal.

A roentgenogram of the skull demonstrated a separation of the sutures as a result of increased intracranial pressure.

A ventriculogram was made. This showed grade 3 symmetric hydrocephalus without any evidence of a space-occupying intracranial lesion. A specimen of cerebrospinal fluid, taken from the ventricles, had a protein content of 180 mg. per 100 cc. Roentgenologic examination of the lumbar and thoracic portions of the spinal column demonstrated scoliosis in the lumbar portion and erosion of the pedicles of the laminae of the thoracic twelfth and the first and second lumbar vertebrae, with enlargement of the spinal canal and thinning of the laminae. The diagnosis was an intraspinal tumor situated between the twelfth thoracic vertebra and the upper border of the third lumbar vertebra.

Differential lumbar puncture was performed at the beginning of the operation but it was not successful because no cerebrospinal fluid could be obtained at the fifth, fourth, and third interspaces; at the second interspace only a few drops of hemorrhagic, xanthochromic cerebrospinal fluid were obtained. A better flow of fluid resulted from puncture done at the twelfth interspace, but complete block was still present at this level. At the eleventh interspace block of the cerebrospinal fluid no longer was present.

Laminectomy was then performed to include the twelfth thoracic through the third lumbar vertebrae. The dura mater was seen to be discolored. An unusually large vessel was present on the dorsal surface of the spinal cord, pushing the conus and the lower part of the dorsal segment of cord upward. A huge tumor (10 by 2 by 2 cm.) was found underneath this vessel. The tumor originated from the filum terminale and extended up and down around the filum terminale and the spinal cord. It had grown into the conus medullaris. All tumor tissue which could be detected grossly was removed. Histologically, the tumor was a grade 1 papillary ependymoma with remarkable endothelial proliferation of the intima of the blood vessels. The dura was closed at the end of the operation.

The postoperative period was uneventful. The papilledema gradually regressed; the headache disappeared. At the time of the patient's dismissal there was only a slight loss of strength in both legs.

Re-examination 2 months later showed marked improvement. The papilledema had completely subsided. The scoliosis in the lumbar area persisted, as did some stiffness of the legs, for which physical therapy was administered at this time.

Two years after removal of the tumor, bone-grafting of the spinal column was done for the scoliosis. At that time it was found that the patient had secondary optic atrophy.

Eleven years after the initial operation the patient was reported to be in good health and to have made no complaints.

Case 8

Nine years before coming to the Mayo Clinic in 1956, a businessman 42 years old began to experience aching pains across both shoulders and in the back. These would be felt only in the early morning, but sometimes they would awaken him from sleep. At times pain also would occur along the entire left arm, sometimes concurrently with, but also sometimes without, the pain in the back. At about this time the patient was seen by several local physicians, but except for extensive psychiatric care no specific treatment was instituted. Several months after the onset of the pain, complete hemianesthesia in respect to pain and temperature developed on the right side of the body. This subsided after a month or two. During the ensuing years the patient continued to experience intermittent pain in the back, shoulder, and left arm.

Seven years after the onset of the pain, numbness developed along the medial aspect of both arms; perception of pain and temperature diminished again, but to a lesser degree than before. Shortly afterward the patient became aware of areas of hyperesthesia over the dorsal aspect of the left arm, and this change was followed by hypesthesia which later changed to hyperesthesia over the abdomen and back. He said that this time he also had noted a "heavy feeling" in his abdomen. Eight years after the onset of the pain he experienced difficulty with orgasm, although erection was normal. He also reported that pain occurred in the groin during intercourse.

Five months before he came to the Mayo Clinic "flexion spasm" developed in the right wrist, and "shaking" in the right leg also was manifest.

Results of a general examination at the Mayo Clinic were negative. Neuromuscular examination disclosed nothing abnormal, but there was a grade 2 hypesthesia which extended over the chest, more marked on the right than on the left, and over part of the shoulders. In addition a moderate degree of analgesia and thermesthesia was found over approximately the same areas. The reflexes in the right arm were slightly elevated, and the Babinski sign was elicited bilaterally. Sense of vibration was almost entirely absent in the legs.

Spinal puncture was performed; complete block of the cerebrospinal circulation was detected. The protein content of the cerebrospinal fluid was 160 mg. per 100 cc.; there were 2 lymphocytes per cubic millimeter of fluid. Results of routine roentgen-ray examination of the cervical and thoracic portions of the spinal column were negative, but a myelogram made with Pantopaque showed complete block of the cephalad flow of the contrast medium at about the level of the second thoracic vertebra.

Laminectomy was performed in which the laminae from the fourth cervical through the third thoracic vertebrae were removed. The dura was found to be tense; after it had been opened, an extensive and large intramedullary tumor could be seen. The posterior columns were split, and after gentle and careful dissection an ependymoma, weighing 48 gm., was removed. The lesion was well encapsulated, but portions of it could be seen descending and ascending in the central axis of the spinal cord. At the end of the operation the dura was left open. Histologically, the tumor was grade 2 mixed ependymoma of the cellular, papillary, and epithelial type.

The postoperative period was uneventful. Roentgen-ray treatment was administered. Examination at the time of dismissal showed that the patient had complete anesthesia over the chest and analgesia which extended over the thighs. At this time all the reflexes were slightly increased; there was minimal loss of strength in the muscles of the hands.

During another examination conducted 15 months after the operation, the patient complained of many difficulties which were, however, not confirmed by the examination. The condition of the patient was found to be essentially the same as at the time of dismissal. After this re-examination the patient received extensive psychiatric treatment for infantile regression with emotional problems.

Four years after the operation the patient's wife said that the patient was gradually becoming worse in every respect. Additional information was gained from the local physician, who said that the symptoms had progressed considerably; paresthesia in the legs and an inability to walk without support were reported. Additional roentgen-ray treatment was suggested.

Case 9

A boy 14 years old had experienced the sudden onset of dull, aching pain in the anterolateral aspect of the right thigh some 15 months before he came to the Mayo Clinic in 1945. The pain was described as "shooting up and down," and was brought on by the patient's sitting or lying down; it was relieved within an hour or two by his walking around. Occasionally the pain would be felt in the same region of the left leg. This pain would be experienced daily to weekly, but it gradually abated during the ensuing summer, approximately 8 months after the onset. Slightly more than a year prior to the beginning of this pain, the patient had sustained a fall on the ice while skating, and the sacrum had been injured. Pain in this region had been present for nearly a year. Ten months before he came to the Mayo Clinic slowing of the stream of urine had developed and 4 months later loss of control of the bladder was complete. Two months later fecal impaction developed which required the daily use of a laxative agent. A roentgenogram made at about this time revealed spina bifida occulta.

When the patient was examined at the Mayo Clinic only a bony deformity over the lower lumbar and sacral region was found. Neurologic examination revealed slight loss of strength in the muscles of the thighs and saddle anesthesia for touch, pain, and temperature. The reflexes were not abnormal, but Babinski's sign was weak bilaterally. Lumbar puncture disclosed nothing abnormal, but the protein content of the cerebrospinal fluid was 220 mg. per 100 cc.

A roentgenogram of the lumbar part of the spinal column revealed a destructive lesion extending from the second lumbar vertebra through the sacral vertebrae, with erosion of the third and fourth sacral segments.

Bilateral laminectomy was performed. After the muscles had been reflected the entire sacrum was found to be bulging. A dark red tumor mass was seen to have eroded through the first, second, third, and fourth sacral segments. The laminae of the fifth lumbar vertebra and the posterior half of the sacrum were removed; this action exposed a tumor mass, the size of a lemon, which extended to the cauda equina. As much of the tumor was removed as was possible. The tumor proved to be a grade 2 myxopapillary ependymoma. During the postoperative course epididymitis developed which was treated successfully.

After the patient was dismissed from the hospital he received a course of roentgen-ray treatment, followed 2 months later by resection of the vesical neck for the incompetence of the sphincter of the bladder. At the time the patient was dismissed he still had saddle anesthesia and slight increase of the tendon reflexes of the legs.

During the ensuing years, the patient occasionally complained of pain in the back and sometimes in the legs, but he could play golf and ping-pong and could ride a scooter. The saddle anesthesia remained consistently present. A roentgenogram made 4 years after the initial operation showed recurrence and extension of the tumor; another course of roentgen-ray treatment was given at this time.

The patient returned again 4 years later, in 1953; examination revealed a slight but definite increase in sensory loss, and a mass could be felt in the hollow of the sacrum. The patient was operated upon again. One centimeter below the surface, on the back, a tumor was found. The eroded laminae of the third and fourth lumbar vertebrae were removed. The incision in the dura was extended to above the upper end of the tumor, and the junction of the tumor with the filum terminale, from which the lesion had taken its origin, could be seen. Extensive removal of the tumor was performed. The postoperative course was notable only because of some drainage from the wound. The operation was followed by another course of roentgen-ray irradiation.

The patient did well for another 2 years, but at the end of that time a non-painful lump was detected at the superior aspect of the surgical scar. Some degree of residual pain was felt in the thighs and calves, and saddle anesthesia for all modalities existed. Moderate weakness of the legs was present. A fourth course of roentgen-ray treatment was given in 1955.

The patient was seen again in 1956. Definite progression of the motor and sensibility symptoms was noted. Eight months after the last visit of the patient to the Mayo Clinic, or 12½ years after the initial operation, word was received that the patient had died at home after an intracranial hemorrhage. Necropsy was reported to have revealed a recurrent ependymoma in the low lumbar and sacral portions of the spinal canal and a metastatic ependymoma attached to the medulla oblongata from which an extensive subarachnoid hemorrhage had originated. Study of histologic sections brought to our attention by Dr. John A. Shively, of Bradenton, Florida, demonstrated tissues of similar structure from lesions in the spinal canal and the medulla oblongata. Both lesions were classified as grade 2 myxopapillary ependymomas, the lesion in the latter situation being a metastatic process in the subdural space, superficially invading the medulla oblongata. No other metastatic processes were found.

Clinical Analysis of Grade 1 and Grade 2 Ependymomas

Our total group of ependymomas consisted of 169 cases. One hundred and eight of these were diagnosed as grade 1, 56 as grade 2 (Table 16), and five as grade 3 ependymoma. Forty of the grade 1 ependymomas were found in the spinal cord itself, and 29 of these were of the cellular type, seven of the epithelial, and four of the papillary type. The remaining 68 in the grade 1 group were found in the filum terminale, and they were classified as follows: cellular type, 27 cases, papillary type, 34 cases, and epithelial type, one case. Six others present in the filum terminale were grouped together as mixed ependymomas, cellular and papillary type. In these cases we were unable to determine the nature of the tumor, since both types were combined.

The 56 grade 2 ependymomas represented nearly a third of all the ependymomas of the spinal cord and the filum terminale in our series. In contrast to what was found in the group of grade 1 ependymomas, there was no predominance of grade 2 lesions in the filum terminale. Half had developed in this structure, and half had arisen in the spinal cord proper. Twenty-six of the tumors of the spinal cord were of the cellular type; the remaining two were classified as mixed ependymomas. One of them contained areas typical of cellular and papillary ependymoma; the other, in addition, contained epithelial areas. Of the 28 tumors of the filum terminale, eight were of the cellular type, 14 of the papillary type, and six of the mixed type.

It is evident that the cellular type of structure is the most frequent in both grade 1 and grade 2 ependymomas. The total of 90 cellular ependymomas constituted more than half of all the lesions in our series. The cellular type was the most frequent tumor of the spinal cord itself, but it represented only approximately a third of all the tumors of the filum terminale. Half of all the tumors of the filum terminale were papillary ependymomas; this type of lesion seems rarely to affect the spinal cord. We had only four instances in our series (Table 16).

Age. At the time of operation the average age (Table 17) of all the patients who had a grade 1 ependymoma was 37 years and 7 months. The youngest patient was 6 years old, and the oldest was 82 years old. Frequency of occurrence of the grade 1 tumor was highest in the fourth decade of life (Table 18); nearly a third, or 37 tumors, had developed in this age group. The average age of patients who had a grade 2 ependymoma was 37 years and 8 months; the youngest patient was 14 years old, and the oldest was 65 years of age. Among those who had grade 2 ependymomas the highest incidence of the lesion was recorded in the fifth decade of life (15 cases) but it was closely followed by the fourth

Table 16. *Classification According to Histologic Type: 164 Ependymomas of Grades 1 and 2*

| | Grade | | | | | | 1 and 2 |
| | 1 | | | 2 | | | |
Type	Cord	Filum	Total	Cord	Filum	Total	Totals
Cellular	29	27	56	26	8	34	90
Papillary	4	34	38	–	14	14	52
Epithelial	7	1	8	–	–	–	8
Mixed	–	6	6	2	6	8	14
Totals	40	68	108	28	28	56	164

Table 17. *Average Age and Sex of Patients: 164 Ependymomas of Grades 1 and 2 Compared on the Basis of Location and Histologic Type*

Lesion, Type, and Location	Grade							
	1				2			
	Cases	Average Age, Yr.	Male	Fe-male	Cases	Average Age, Yr.	Male	Fe-male
Total group	108	37 7/12	66	42	56	37 8/12	30	26
Spinal cord	40	43 4/12	25	15	28	40	14	14
Filum terminale	68	34 3/12	41	27	28	35 3/12	16	12
Cellular, cord	29	45 7/12	20	9	26	39 11/12	13	13
Cellular, filum terminale	27	36	13	14	8	40 3/12	4	4
Papillary, cord	4	32 6/12	2	2	–	–	–	–
Papillary, filum terminale	34	33 9/12	24	10	14	34 3/12	9	5
Epithelial, cord	7	40 5/12	3	4	–	–	–	–
Epithelial, filum terminale	1	51	1	–	–	–	–	–
Mixed, cord	–	–	–	–	2	42	1	1
Mixed, filum terminale	6	26 10/12	3	3	6	30 10/12	3	3

(13 cases). In Figure 15 the incidence, according to decades of age of the patients, of 169 ependymomas, 86 astrocytomas, 376 neurilemmomas, and 337 meningiomas is seen.

When the average age of patients who have tumors of the spinal cord is compared with that of patients who have similar tumors of the filum terminale, a remarkable difference becomes apparent: the average age of the patient who had a grade 1 ependymoma of the spinal cord was 43 years and 4 months, whereas the average age of the patient who had a grade 1 ependymoma of the filum terminale was 34 years and 3 months (Table 17). In the case of patients who had grade 2 ependymomas of the spinal cord, the average age was 40 years, whereas among those who had grade 2 ependymomas of the filum terminale the average age was 35 years and 3 months. Further analysis (Table 17) would seem to indicate that grade 1 cellular ependymomas of the filum terminale, as well as papillary ependymomas of grades 1 and 2 situated in the cord and filum terminale, occur at an average younger age of the patient than do tumors in other groups. Our series is rather small for statistical comparisons, however, and for this reason analysis of small groups within the series probably is of questionable benefit.

Table 18. Frequency of Occurrence, by Decades, of 169 Ependymomas of Grades 1 to 3

Age, Years	Grade 1	Grade 2	Grade 3	Totals No.	Totals Per Cent
0 – 9	1	–	–	1	0.7
10 – 19	9	7	1	17	10.0
20 – 29	18	9	–	27	16.0
30 – 39	37	13	1	51	30.1
40 – 49	20	15	–	35	20.7
50 – 59	18	10	–	28	16.5
60 – 69	3	2	2	7	4.1
70 – 79	1	–	1	2	1.2
80 + over	1	–	–	1	0.7
Totals	108	56	5	169	100.0

Sex. Sixty-one per cent of the grade 1 ependymomas and 54 per cent of the grade 2 ependymomas occurred in males. This confirms the general impression that the occurrence of gliomas is slightly more frequent in males. Review of the subgroups in Table 17 in general confirms the impression of a predominance for the male sex.

Location and Extent of the Lesions. As already has been mentioned, nearly two-thirds of grade 1 ependymomas and one-half of grade 2 ependymomas were found in the filum terminale. This minute structure also accounts for more than half of all the ependymomas. If the data in Table 19 are compared with the data in Table 4 having to do with the expected incidence based on the vertebral level, it becomes evident that, in our series, the incidence of ependymomas in the thoracic area was much lower (16.3 per cent), and that the incidence of ependymomas in the lumbar area (28.5 per cent) was higher than the expected incidences of tumors of the spinal cord (51.5 per cent and 26 per cent, respectively [Table 4]).

The length, or size, of the lesions, based on the extent of the laminectomy, was variable. In several instances the length of an ependymoma extended over 10 vertebrae. The average length, however, was much shorter: 59 of the grade 1 ependymomas necessitated laminectomy involving three to five vertebrae, and in all but five cases grade 2 ependymomas required laminectomy involving two to six vertebrae. In Figure 44 the location and length of the individual lesions, on the basis of the extent of the laminectomy required, are given.

Preoperative Duration. The average preoperative duration of symptoms among patients who had grade 1 ependymomas was 56 months; this period was 33 months among those who had grade 2 ependymomas. In Table 20 detailed analysis of the particular types and locations of lesions has been made, from which it appears that the duration of symptoms among patients who had grade 1 papillary ependymomas located in the filum terminale was longer than the duration of symptoms

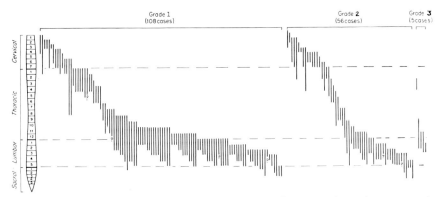

Figure 44. Anatomic location and extension of 169 instances of ependymoma, grade 1 to grade 3.

Table 19. *Frequency of Occurrence of 164 Ependymomas According to Vertebral Level and Histologic Type*

Level, Vertebral	Cellular		Papillary		Epithelial		Mixed		Totals			
	Grade										1 and 2	
	1	2	1	2	1	2	1	2	1	2	No.	Per Cent
Cervical	7	12	–	–	2	–	–	1	8	14	22	13.3
Cervicothoracic	2	3	–	–	4	–	–	1	6	4	10	6.1
Thoracic	14	9	3	–	1	–	–	–	18	9	27	16.3
Thoracolumbar	17	5	16	4	–	–	2	1	34	11	45	27.3
Lumbar	14	3	14	8	1	–	4	3	33	14	47	28.5
Lumbosacral	3	1	3	2	–	–	–	2	6	5	11	7.3
Sacral	–	–	2	–	–	–	–	–	2	–	2	1.2

Table 20. *Preoperative Duration of Symptoms and Postoperative Survival: 159 Patients Who Had Ependymomas of Grades 1 and 2, Based on Histologic Type and Location*

	Grade 1				Grade 2			
	Duration							
	Preoperative		Postoperative		Preoperative		Postoperative	
Lesion, Type, Location	No.	Months	No.	Months	No.	Months	No.	Months
Total group	105	56	95	151	54	33	46	111
Spinal cord	39	52	35	114	27	49	22	124
Filum terminale	66	58	60	173	27	17	24	99
Cellular type, cord	29	56	24	118	25	47	20	134
Cellular type, filum terminale	26	61	26	174	7	18	7	63
Papillary type, cord	4	20	4	150	–	–	–	–
Papillary type, filum terminale	34	62	30	178	14	16	11	114
Epithelial type, cord	6	55	7	81	–	–	–	–
Epithelial type, filum terminale	–	–	–	–	–	–	–	–
Mixed type, cord	–	–	–	–	2	78	2	30
Mixed type, filum terminale	6	28	4	126	6	17	6	111

among patients who had the same type of tumor located in the spinal cord. A similar but less marked parallelism in duration of symptoms is noted among patients who had the cellular type of ependymoma, viewed from the standpoint of location in the cord as opposed to location in the filum terminale.

Variation in the preoperative duration among the individual patients ranged from 6 weeks to 20 years, but in almost two-thirds of all patients the duration of symptoms was 4 years or less, and in only 14 patients was the duration 10 years or more.

Postoperative Survival.   The average postoperative survival of all patients who had grade 1 ependymomas was 151 months, whereas that of patients who had grade 2 ependymomas was 111 months (Table 20). Survival of patients who had a grade 1 tumor in the spinal cord was shorter (114 months) than that of patients who had a grade 1 ependymoma in the filum terminale (173 months). Remarkably enough, the opposite was true among patients who had grade 2 lesions; the survival among those who had lesions of the spinal cord was 124 months, whereas among those who had tumors of the filum terminale the survival was 99 months. Among those who had grade 1 cellular ependymomas of the spinal cord the survival was 118 months; among those who had this lesion in the filum terminale, the survival was 174 months (Table 20). Again there was a reversal in respect to grade 2 cellular ependymomas: among patients who had these lesions in the spinal cord, the survival was 134 months; among those whose lesions were situated in the filum terminale the survival was only 63 months (Table 20). As for the remaining lesions—papillary, epithelial, and mixed types—it was found, as would be expected, that among patients who had the more malignant tumors the survival was shorter.

We are not able to offer a satisfactory explanation for the contradictory lengths of survival among patients who had the cellular types of ependymomas, although we are aware of several factors which might have exerted some influence. That is, from one aspect, the averages given in Table 20 represent minimal periods of time in the sense that some of the patients were still alive at the time of our study. For instance, among those who had grade 1 ependymomas, in 93 instances it was known whether the patient was alive or dead. In the event of latter occurrence, the year after operation in which the patient died also was known. In Table 21 it will be seen that 54 of 93 patients who had had grade 1 ependymomas were alive at the time of this study, and that 39 had been reported to be dead, producing a survival rate of 58 per cent. Of the 48 patients who had had grade 2 ependymomas, 26 were known to be alive and 22 had died, producing a survival rate of 54 per cent (Table 21).

Consideration also must be given to the extent of the therapy. In Table 22 a comparison is made between the types of surgical treatment

Table 21.   *Five-Year Survival Periods: 131 Patients Who Had Ependymomas of Grades 1 and 2*

Period, Years	Grade 1				Grade 2			
	Cord		Filum		Cord		Filum	
	Dead	Living	Dead	Living	Dead	Living	Dead	Living
< 5	14	4	10	5	7	3	8	4
5 - 9	4	4	2	3	3	3	–	3
10 - 14	–	2	2	12	1	1	2	2
15 - 19	2	4	1	10	–	4	–	2
20 - 24	1	1	–	5	–	3	1	1
25 - 29	1	–	1	–	–	–	–	–
30 or more	–	–	1	4	–	–	–	–
Totals	22	15	17	39	11	14	11	12

performed, whether with or without roentgen-ray irradiation, and the length of survival and percentage of surviving patients, among 138 who had grade 1 and grade 2 ependymomas. Interpretation of the data in this table must be done very carefully, for several reasons. First, it will be noticed that some of the subgroups are extremely small, consisting of only one or two cases. Second, a variable number of patients in the several categories were still alive, at varying intervals after operation, at the time our study was made. Hence the data in Table 22 are by no means final. Third, roentgen-ray treatment in a number of instances had been administered elsewhere, as a rule not under our supervision, which means that we do not know how much roentgen-ray irradiation was given or how adequately it was administered. In addition, slightly more patients who had grade 2 lesions received roentgen-ray treatment than did patients who had grade 1 lesions (45 per cent).

The percentage of survival sustains fairly well the assumption that the more extensive the treatment is, the better the prognosis will be. That the survival time in our series did not sustain this assumption perhaps might be accounted for, at least partially, by the fact that at the time the study was made, more patients were still alive in each of the categories in which treatment had been more extensive. It would appear from the data in Table 23, that on the average, the postoperative

Table 22. *Survival Time and Percentage of Survival of 138 Patients With Ependymomas in Relation to the Extent and Nature of the Therapy*

Treatment, Type	Grade 1								Grade 2							
	Spinal Cord				Filum Terminale				Spinal Cord				Filum Terminale			
	No.	Average Survival, Months	Alive No.	Per Cent	No.	Average Survival, Months	Alive No.	Per Cent	No.	Average Survival, Months	Alive No.	Per Cent	No.	Average Survival, Months	Alive No.	Per Cent
Total removal					28	196	23	82	3	200	1	33	8	141	5	63
Subtotal removal	12	124	7	58	6	65	2	33	4	138	2	50	4	62	2	50
Biopsy	5	154	0	0					2	23	0	0	1	30	0	0
Total removal and roentgen rays	2	78	2	100	13	164	11	85	1	300	1	100	6	114	4	66
Subtotal removal and roentgen rays	11	127	5	45	11	177	10	90	10	119	8	80	4	53	1	25
Biopsy and roentgen rays	4	47	2	50	1	228	0	0	1	24	1	100	1	12	0	0

Table 23. *Survival Time of 128 Patients With Ependymomas, Grades 1 and 2, in Relation to Their Location in the Spinal Cord*

Location of Lesion	Grade			
	1		2	
	No.	Survival, Months	No.	Survival, Months
Cervical	8	105	9	141
Cervicothoracic	5	93	4	71
Thoracic	14	108	7	108
Thoracolumbar	32	178	9	122
Lumbar	22	156	11	114
Lumbosacral	3	92	4	62

survival of patients who had ependymomas in the cervical area was not any shorter than the survival of those who had ependymomas in the thoracic area. Actually, when grade 2 ependymomas are considered, patients whose lesions developed in the cervical area, with an average survival time of 141 months, did even better than patients whose lesions were located in any other segment of the spinal cord (Table 23).

Lack of a clear difference in the matter of survival times between patients who had grade 1 tumors and patients who had grade 2 tumors is not surprising, in view of the unusual behavior of cellular ependymomas, which constitute most grade 2 tumors of the spinal cord.

We mention the additional factor that in a certain number of cases diagnosis was made only on material that had been taken for biopsy, and we are fully aware of the diagnostic insufficiency of such a procedure.

Another point which should be considered in this respect is the cause of death. We are not completely informed on this point in relation to our series, since most of the patients died elsewhere. Cases in which necropsy was performed at the Mayo Clinic will be described in more detail in Chapter IV. Information which we obtained in the remaining cases indicates that nearly all patients died of the indirect results of tumors of the spinal cord. Among these indirect effects infection of the bladder and kidney (pyelonephritis and hydronephrosis) appears to have been the most important. Many of the patients who had this complication died before the era of chemotherapeutic and antibiotic agents, but even currently the complication represents a serious problem which often ultimately causes the death of the patient, although the period of survival may be lengthened. Another serious problem is the development of decubital or trophic ulcers, which can result in septicemia or erosion of a blood vessel. This complication also can be influenced favorably by modern therapeutic methods. In a very few cases we have been able to prove that death resulted from metastasis of a tumor of the spinal cord, and in a few other cases there was a strong suggestion of metastasis.

Some of the patients died of totally unrelated causes which include such conditions as carcinoma of the cervix uteri, tuberculosis, and arteriosclerotic dementia.

Subjective symptoms which suggested recurrence or progression of the tumor were found in about a fourth of our cases. In six patients (or 5.5 per cent) who had a grade 1 ependymoma and in nine patients (or 18 per cent) who had a grade 2 ependymoma, recurrence or progression of the lesion necessitated a second operation. In a few additional cases roentgen-ray irradiation was administered instead.

One patient was unusual in the sense that his recurrent tumor was of grade 1 malignancy, whereas the lesion found at the time of the first operation had been judged to be of grade 2 malignancy.

Symptoms.   The first symptom of 82 of the 107 patients who had a grade 1 ependymoma and of 35 of the patients who had a grade 2 ependymoma was pain. Of these 117 patients, 60 indicated that the pain was in the back, nine said that the pain occurred in the back and in one or both lower extremities, and 16 said that the pain was felt in the legs only; six patients experienced pain in the thorax, groin, or interscapular region; eight reported pain in the neck, and six said pain had been felt in the arms.

Three patients said that the first symptom of a tumor was "rectal discomfort."

Twenty-one patients reported that a sensory disturbance, generally described as "numbness," hypesthesia, or a sensation of coldness, was the first symptom. The disturbance was located in the leg in nine patients, in the arms in seven, in the trunk in four, and in the buttocks in one.

Motor dysfunction, described as a first symptom, was said to have been present in 15 patients. It was found 10 times in the legs, three times in the arms, and twice in the neck.

Five patients said the first symptom they noticed was difficulty in urination or in bowel movements or the development of impotence.

When the patients were first seen at the Mayo Clinic 135 complained of pain which could be related to the presence of a tumor in the spinal cord or filum terminale. Pain of this type seemed to be less constant in patients who had a tumor of the spinal cord. Forty patients (59 per cent) with a tumor in the spinal cord complained of pain of this kind, whereas pain was present in all but one of the patients who had a tumor of the filum terminale.

During physical examination 36 patients reported that pain was the only symptom, except for some minor reflex changes.

An additional 99 patients said that pain was present with varying combinations of motor or sensory dysfunction and disturbances of the bladder or bowel. Thirteen patients reported a combination of pain and motor symptoms; nine others spoke of pain and sensory symptoms. Forty-eight patients had, in addition to pain, motor and sensory disturbances and another 22 had, in addition to the foregoing, sphincter incompetence.

Three patients had, in addition to dysfunction of the bladder or bowel, pain and sensory impairment; two others had pain and motor incapacity; and two had only pain in addition to the sphincter disturbance.

One hundred and four patients had some form of sensory dysfunction. In addition to combinations with pain which have just been mentioned, sensory dysfunction was the only symptom of one patient; 12 others had, in addition, associated motor dysfunction. Another nine had motor and bladder dysfunction in addition to sensory impairment.

Muscle function was affected in 108 patients. In two patients this difficulty was the only symptom; as we have said previously, 13 patients had the combination of pain and motor dysfunction. Forty-eight patients had, in addition to pain and motor dysfunction, sensory disturbance; two others had, in addition to pain and motor impairment, difficulties with the bladder or bowel. Twenty-two more had sensory impairment as well as pain, motor dysfunction, and difficulty with the bladder or the bowel. Twelve patients had the combination of motor and sensory impairment, and nine others had difficulties with sphincters.

Disturbance of the function of bladder and bowel was present as a symptom in 40 patients; this type of disturbance appears to have been slightly more prominent among persons who had tumors of the filum terminale than it was among those who had tumors of the spinal cord. In no patient was this type of disturbance the only symptom, and when it was present it was always accompanied by other manifestations. Changes in reflexes, such as either accentuation or diminution of the tendon reflexes, were found to be present in all except 28 cases.

Cerebrospinal Fluid.   Lumbar puncture had been performed for 118 patients who had a grade 1 or a grade 2 ependymoma; in 10 cases "dry tap" was encountered. In 59 patients who had grade 1 ependymomas the content of protein in the cerebrospinal fluid was determined; the average value in this group was 2157 mg. per 100 cc. Among patients who had tumors of the spinal cord the protein content averaged 542 mg. per 100 cc., and among those who had tumors of the filum terminale the protein content was 3144 mg. per 100 cc. Among 45 patients who

had grade 2 ependymomas the average content of protein in the cerebrospinal fluid was 1100 mg. per 100 cc.; among those who had tumors of
the spinal cord it was 852 mg. per 100 cc.; and among patients who had
tumors of the filum terminale the protein content was 1358 mg. per
100 cc. of fluid.

In only seven patients—five with a tumor of the spinal cord and two
with a tumor of the filum terminale—was the protein content of the
cerebrospinal fluid within the normal range (meaning less than 40 mg.
per 100 cc..); in 21 patients (14 with tumors of the cord and seven with
tumors of the filum terminale) it ranged between 40 and 100 mg. per
100 cc.; in 47 patients (20 with tumors of the cord and 27 with tumors
of the filum terminale) it ranged between 100 and 1000 mg. per 100 cc.,
and in 29 patients (six with tumors of the cord and 23 with tumors of
the filum terminale) the protein content was more than 1000 mg. per 100
cc. of fluid.

In 50 patients partial or total block of the cerebrospinal fluid was
found (not considered in this group are the 10 patients in whom dry tap
was encountered). A detailed analysis of the average values for protein
in the cerebrospinal cord in relation to the presence or absence of partial
or total block is found in Table 24. As might be expected, the protein
content increased as obstruction of the flow of cerebrospinal fluid
increased.

The average number of cells in the cerebrospinal fluid was 5 to 6 per
cubic millimeter. In the matter of cell content of the cerebrospinal fluid,

*Table 24. Average Content of Protein in the Cerebrospinal Fluid Cor-
related With Degree of Obstruction of Fluid: 104 Patients*
With Ependymomas of Grades 1 and 2 in Whom the
Protein Content Was Determined*

	Lesion, Grade						
	1				2		
	Spinal Cord		Filum Terminale		Spinal Cord		Filum Terminale	
Cerebrospinal Fluid Condition	No.	Average Protein, mg., %	No.	Average Protein, mg., %	No.	Average Protein, mg., %	No.	Average Protein, mg., %
No block	11	370	19	2665	8	130	16	1005
Partial block	3	81	2	2950	3	90	1	500
Total block	8	952	16	3706	12	1532	5	2664

*Lumbar puncture performed in 118 patients; results available
concerning 104.

there appeared to be no significance in location of the tumor in the spinal cord or location in the filum terminale, nor any significance in whether block of the cerebrospinal fluid was or was not present.

Roentgenograms and Myelography.   Plain roentgenograms were helpful to the diagnosis in only 14 patients who had grade 1 ependymomas and in 11 who had grade 2 ependymomas. In these instances it showed erosion of the pedicles or widening of the spinal canal which appeared to be indicative of a tumor of the spinal cord.

A myelogram made with radiopaque oil was obtained in 64 cases; it disclosed nothing of significance in two patients found to have a tumor of the filum terminale, and it gave information of doubtful value in four additional patients.

In addition to observations which leave no doubt of the presence of a tumor of the spinal cord, a few other observations seem worthy of mention, although their relationship to tumors of the spinal cord or of the filum terminale is doubtful or unknown. Sixteen patients had an anatomic malformation of the vertebrae. This malformation ranged from spina bifida in nine, spondylolisthesis in two, sacralization of the lumbar vertebrae in two, presence of only four lumbar vertebrae in one, and wedging and compression of a vertebra in two. In another 10 cases scoliosis or kyphoscoliosis was noted.

The significance of the presence of papilledema has been discussed in Chapter I, "Symptomatologic Factors," p. 15. This condition was present three times in the total series of patients with ependymomas.

In 32 patients the surgeon noticed during the operation cavitation of the spinal cord at a site near the tumor. In 16 of these cases we found histologic evidence suggestive of syringomyelia.

Grade 3 Ependymoma.   Only five lesions were classified as grade 3 ependymomas. One of them was a papillary type; a second one showed focal areas with papillary structures. The remaining three tumors were of the cellular type, although one of them had an occasional area with an epithelial arrangement.

The average age of these five patients was 49 years and 5 months; however, three patients were more than 60 years old, and the youngest one was 11 years old. Three were females, and two were males.

One of the tumors was located in the thoracic area from the second to the fourth thoracic vertebrae; the remaining four tumors were found in the filum terminale.

The average preoperative period was 8 months, a period which is much shorter than that of patients who had lesions of the other two lower grades. The shortest duration of symptoms was one month, and the longest, 17 months. Three patients had symptoms which were present 7 months or less.

The postoperative survival periods were variable. One patient, 76 years of age, died 8 months after the subtotal removal of a tumor from the filum terminale. The second patient died 38 months after subtotal removal of a grade 3 ependymoma from the area of the second to the fourth thoracic vertebrae. The third patient was known to be alive 11 months after total removal of a tumor which had originated from the filum terminale. The fourth patient was alive 5 years after removal of a similar tumor, but this patient also had received a course of roentgen-ray treatment. This patient also was known to have progressive paralysis of the legs, and at the time of this report she was confined to a wheelchair. The fifth patient was lost to our records 5 years after total removal of an ependymoma of the filum terminale. He had undergone another operation 9 months after removal of the ependymoma, at which time decompression had been carried out.

The symptoms manifested by patients who had grade 3 ependymomas were not dissimilar to those of patients with lesions in other groups, although the development of the symptoms was more rapid than it was in other categories. Syringomyelia was found in one patient at necropsy. Details concerning these patients can be found in the appendix.

OLIGODENDROGLIOMAS

In our series there were eight tumors which were derived from oligodendroglia.

It is said that Robertson was the first to recognize the oligodendroglial cell. He distinguished it from the group of "dwarf satellites" or "third element" of Cajal. He thought that these cells are of mesodermal origin, and he therefore called them "mesoglia."

In 1924 Bailey and Hiller[17] translated part of the original work of Santiago Ramón y Cajal and his pupils, Pio del Rio Hortega and Nicolás Achucárro, into English and brought this important work to the attention and benefit of others. The latter two Spanish authors were able, with the aid of their special staining technics, to recognize the oligodendroglial cell among the third element of Cajal.

The oligodrendroglial cell was described as having a spherical and rather vesicular nucleus which, in the matter of size and density of the chromatin network, would range somewhere between the nuclei of microglia and the nuclei of neuroglia. The cytoplasm forms a finely granular mass which may be rounded but often is polygonal and is said usually to be eccentrically located in relation to the nucleus. Often the cytoplasm stains only faintly or not at all, with ordinary staining methods. The cells possess slender, delicate, dichotomously branching processes which taper rapidly to an even caliber and show small enlargements at irregular intervals, in the center of which a vacuole may be seen after Hortega's silver-impregnation method has been used.

The cells are found, for the most part, in long rows along the fiber tracts of the brain and in the spinal cord. In the gray matter they appear to be almost exclusively satellites which are present near the base of the neurons.

In the study of Bailey and Hiller[17] (1924), as in the study of Bailey and Cushing[16] (1926), the existence of oligodendrogliomas is indicated and a few examples are described, but it was not until 1929 that Bailey and Bucy[14] could prove that certain tumors in the nervous system are derived from this cell type.

The tumors are described as being exceedingly cellular, and the cells are said to be remarkably uniform. The nuclei are almost perfectly round; they have a fairly constant size and are regularly distributed throughout the tumor. The cytoplasm is described as being very indistinct and, when it was visible with the ordinary staining methods, it was finely granular and eosinophilic. Individual cells are separated from each other by fibrillary intercellular material. The tumors are likely to exhibit many areas in which there are typical, swollen, oligodendroglial cells. These cells have small, dark-staining nuclei located in the center of optically clear or only faintly pink-staining cytoplasm which is surrounded by a heavily impregnated cellular membrane. Other features are the rarity of mitotic figures, the moderate vascularity, and the common occurrence of endothelial proliferation in the blood vessels.

Typical also of oligodendrogliomas are areas of calcification which, in most cases in our series, were grossly apparent.

In 1932 one of us (Kernohan)[141] made a further attempt to define oligodendrogliomatous types by suggesting the possibility of a subgroup, the oligodendroblastomas, in which cells have larger nuclei and in which the cytoplasm is more readily visible. In these tumors mitosis was more frequent.

Earnest, Craig, and one of us [Kernohan[71] (1950)] were unable to obtain a correlation between the histologic appearance and the life history of oligodendroglial tumors similar to that which forms the basis for the system of grading astrocytomas and ependymomas. Even classification of the tumors as oligodendrogliomas and oligodendroblastomas on the basis of the microscopic examination seemed to lose significance when applied to the survival period. Still, it was judged to be reasonable to anticipate a longer period of survival for patients who have oligodendrogliomas.

The frequency of occurrence of oligodendrogliomas in the spinal cord appears to be very low. Only six cases are known to us [Oljenick[205] (1936); Gagel[100] (1938); Woods-Pimenta[309] (1944); Russell-Bucy[247] (1949); Eneström-Gröntoft[85] (1957)].

Gross (Figs. 45 and 46)

In the available descriptions of gross specimens the color of oligodendrogliomas ranges from red to purple to brown. The gross appearance

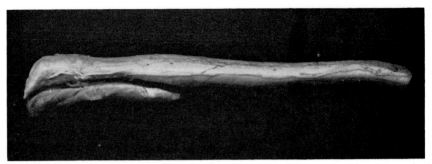

Figure 45. An oligodendroglioma originating from the anterior side of the spinal cord and extending into the subarachnoid space in case 32 in Chapter IV. See also Figure 46.

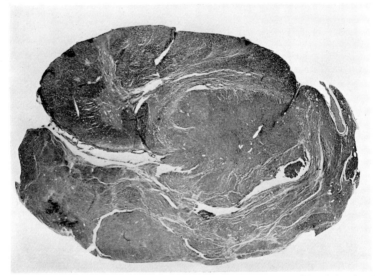

Figure 46. Oligodendroglioma, same case as in Figure 45, originating from the anterior side of the cord and extending into the subarachnoid space (hematoxylin and eosin; × 5).

is granular. We found no feature which would distinguish these tumors from astrocytomas or ependymomas. In two cases cysts were described in relationship to the tumor.

Histologic Aspects

In histologic features oligodendroglioma is cellular and fairly monotonous. The nuclei are of moderate size; many are spherical but others are oval or slightly polygonal. The chromatin content is fairly dense, and the chromatin often appears as fine, dustlike particles which as a rule are regularly dispersed over the karyoplasm. Sometimes the chromatin may be coarser or it may be assembled below the nuclear membrane, giving the nucleus a vesicular appearance. Careful examination often reveals

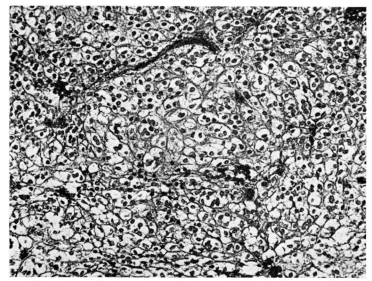

Figure 47. Oligodendroglioma. The nuclei have a clear halo and the cellular borders appear prominent (hematoxylin and eosin; × 250).

slight pleomorphism as indicated by the presence of a few slightly larger, irregular-shaped nuclei. Nucleoli can be found in a number of nuclei; we noted the presence of inclusion bodies in several tumors, but such an observation was infrequent.

The nuclei are distributed regularly throughout the tumor, and often are placed in a fairly wide, clear area (Fig. 47) which is surrounded by a heavily impregnated membrane. Frequently, a few faintly staining granules, arranged in fine bands, are seen in the otherwise optically clear cytoplasm. Other nuclei are located in a pale pink, sometimes slightly granular, cytoplasm which is also clearly demarcated. In both cellular variations the nucleus is fairly often, but need not be, centrally located.

The cells are closely packed. We were usually unable to distinguish any intercellular substance. There is no prominent cellular form, since the cells adjust their form to the mosaic pattern. The areas, for the most part composed of clear cells, have an unusual appearance which resembles that of a plantlike structure or which has a honeycomb appearance (Fig. 48). No other architectural structure could be detected. The vascularity of oligodendrogliomas is variable; we found that some were very vascular, and others were much less so. Some endothelial swelling and proliferation were seen, but they appeared to be of a minor degree. The tumor cells did not have a specific arrangement around the vessels.

In none of the tumors did we see calcification or areas of necrosis, although these are said to be frequent accompaniments of oligodendrogliomas of the brain.

Oligodendroblastomas are distinguished by a more marked irregularity

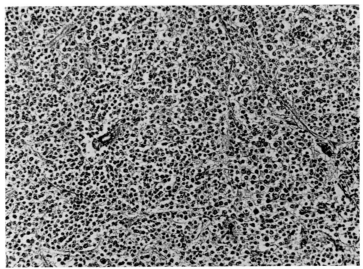

Figure 48. Oligodendroglioma presenting a monotonous honeycomb or plantlike picture (hematoxylin and eosin; × 175).

and pleomorphism of the nuclei, which also are generally somewhat larger than the nuclei of oligodendrogliomas. The content and appearance of chromatin in the oligodendroblastomas remain approximately the same, as in oligodendrogliomas, but mitotic figures are more frequent. There is less of a tendency for the cells to present a swollen, honeycomb-like appearance, and sometimes it is even difficult to distinguish cytoplasm around the nuclei. When the cytoplasm is present about the nuclei it stains faintly pink and is seen to be granular. In a number of cells it is clearly outlined. The vascularity remains variable, but vascular reactions in the form of proliferation and swelling of the endothelial cells are more frequently identified. There were no areas of necrosis, and we did not see calcification.

In one of the oligodendrogliomas were areas which were indistinguishable from areas in the cellular type of ependymoma. In those fields a clear perivascular arrangement was seen.

Clinical Aspects

In our series eight tumors were derived from the oligodendroglia. Of these, five were judged to be oligodendrogliomas, and three, oligodendroblastomas. Only one of the total group, an oligodendroglioma, was found in the filum terminale; all the others were found in the spinal cord.

Age.   The average age of all the patients who had a tumor of this type was 37 years and 9 months; the oldest was 52, and the youngest, 19 years of age. There is no remarkable difference between the average age of patients who have oligodendroglioma and the average age of patients who have oligodendroblastoma.

Sex.   Five males and three females were affected.

Location.   Three of the tumors, one oligodendroglioma and two oligodendroblastomas, were present in the cervical portion of the spinal cord. Three oligodendrogliomas were found in the thoracic portion of the spinal cord; one oligodendroblastoma developed in the conus medullaris; and one oligodendroglioma was located in the filum terminale.

Extension of the lesions varied between two and five vertebral levels.

Preoperative Duration.   Among the seven patients in this group the average preoperative duration of lesions was 21 months. One case, in which the preoperative duration was 10 years, is outstanding. The shortest preoperative duration of symptoms was 7 months.

Postoperative Duration.   Only two of the eight patients were known to be alive at the time of this report. Both had undergone what was thought to be complete removal of the tumor; one of them, who had survived for 29 years at the time of the last report, had had a clearly encapsulated tumor between the fourth and fifth cervical levels. She also had received a course of roentgen-ray therapy. The other patient was alive 22 years after removal of the tumor of the filum terminale. This last patient was reported to be in excellent health, but the former had some residual numbness and pain in the left hand.

The fate of one patient is unknown; she had an oligodendroblastoma of the conus medullaris. At the time of operation this had extended and appeared to be infiltrating the nerve roots of the cauda equina. The remaining patients are known to be dead. One of them died 6 years and 4 months after the first subtotal removal of an oligodendroglioma at the level of the eighth to eleventh thoracic vertebrae. He also had received a course of roentgen-ray therapy. About 5 years after the operation, blurred vision, paraplegia, papilledema, and anesthesia extending up to the ninth thoracic level developed. Subtotal removal of a recurrent oligodendroglioma was done. The patient died at home 16 months later. Necropsy was reported to have disclosed a recurrent oligodendroglioma in the spinal cord, and there were meningeal lesions at the inferior surface of the cerebellum, brain stem, and interpeduncular region; these lesions were described by the local pathologist as being composed of "undifferentiated spongioblasts."

The second patient died 30 months after biopsy and decompression of the spinal cord between the third and seventh cervical vertebrae. The tumor was identified as an oligodendroblastoma.

The third patient died approximately 24 months after a specimen for biopsy had been taken from an oligodendroglioma extending from the fourth to the eighth thoracic vertebrae. During the last week of life the vision of the patient failed and deafness developed; there was marked papilledema. Necropsy was performed elsewhere than at the Mayo Clinic; the brain was reported as being normal. The spinal cord was sent to us, and the findings will be discussed in Chapter IV (case 33).

The last patient died 3 weeks after total removal of what was thought to be a dumbbell neurofibroma. At necropsy an intramedullary oligo-dendroblastoma was found in the cervical portion of the spinal cord. The detailed findings are given in Chapter IV (case 32).

Symptoms.   All eight patients reported pain to be the first sign of the tumor. In all except one case the pain was located in a region of the back. In the one exception the pain was felt in the left quadriceps muscle.

Neurologic examination of six patients revealed a combined disturb-ance of motor and sensory functions; in one patient only motor dysfunc-tion was found. Results of examination of the last patient were negative except for some reflex changes.

In five patients complete or partial block of the cerebrospinal fluid was noted at the time of lumbar puncture. The protein content of the cere-brospinal fluid was recorded in five patients; it varied from 160 to 5000 mg. per 100 cc. of fluid. The highest cell count in the group was 10 per cubic millimeter of fluid. Details can be found in the tables at the end of this book.

Roentgen-ray examination was found to be diagnostic of a tumor of the spinal cord in two patients. In one, destruction of a vertebra was seen, and in the second—the one previously mentioned as suspected of having a dumbbell neurofibroma—widening of the root canal was detected.

A myelogram was made in two instances, and results were positive in both.

MIXED GLIOMAS

Among the astrocytomas, as well as the ependymomas, we found cell groups which resembled the cells of an oligodendroglioma. But in one oligodendroglioma we found an area which exhibited the typical cells and structures of an ependymoma. It is, therefore, not surprising to learn that we found three tumors in which two tumor types were so extensively intermixed that we felt it justified in calling the tumors "mixed gliomas."

The combination of astrocytes and oligodendrocytes was described in 1929 by Bailey and Bucy,[14] and in 1937 Fletcher-Kernohan and one of us (Kernohan) [144] called attention to the frequent intermingling of oligo-dendrocytes in ependymomas.

In two patients, both females, 18 and 40 years of age, the tumor was located in the filum terminale. The histologic structure was a mixture of areas typical of cellular ependymoma and oligodendroglioma. Some-times these areas were intermixed, sometimes they were sharply demar-cated from each other, and sometimes they were separated by a zone of tumor tissue which was difficult to identify. The malignancy of both components appeared to be low. The surgical attack on both tumors was total removal. One was described as being 20 cm. long; the other was 6 cm. long and 3 to 4 cm. in width.

The clinical symptoms in both cases were similar to those caused by other gliomas.

The first patient, 40 years old, complained of backache that had begun after an automobile accident. The backache had been present for 15 years. Many years later weakness of the legs had developed gradually, but sensation was normal at the time of examination. Roentgenologic examination disclosed erosion of the first three lumbar vertebrae. After the operation, the patient received a course of roentgen-ray treatment, and she was still living 19 years after the operation. Her neurologic status was unknown to us at the time of this report.

The second patient, 18 years old, reported pain in the posterior aspect of the right thigh that had begun 3½ months prior to the operation. At examination sensory disturbance was noted in both thighs and buttocks and in the perianal region. Motor function was normal, but both achilles reflexes were graded —4. A myelogram made with Pantopaque revealed complete block of the oil at the level of the first sacral vertebra. What was thought to be total removal of the tumor was performed. Four months after this operation, the symptoms recurred and another operation was performed, 8 months after the first one. Nothing definite could be found at the second operation. A Pantopaque myelogram made 2½ months after this procedure revealed complete block at the level of the second lumbar vertebra. At the third operation a recurrent tumor of the filum terminale was totally removed. The patient received a course of roentgen-ray treatment after this operation and did reasonably well for 11 years, but recurrence was noted again and another operation was done elsewhere than at the Mayo Clinic. The patient was still alive 19 years after the initial operation, and was married and had three children at the time of this report. She needed, however, constant care for infections of the bladder and kidneys and daily laxative agents to overcome constipation.

The third patient was a girl 20 years old. She had pain across the chest that she had first noticed 2 months before she was operated upon; this pain was soon followed by sensations of tingling and numbness in the right hand and arm. Examination also demonstrated loss of strength in both arms. At lumbar puncture, complete block was found. The protein content of the cerebrospinal fluid was 7500 mg. per 100 cc. At operation what was thought to be complete removal was accomplished of a tumor located at the level of the first thoracic vertebra. Her neurologic status did not improve, and she was reported to have died 2 months later.

Histologic examination of the tumor revealed that it was composed of areas of a grade 2 astrocytoma intermixed with an oligodendroblastoma.

III

Nongliomatous Tumors

In this category we assembled a heterogeneous group of neoplasms which have the common features that they were found inside the substance of the spinal cord, that evidence was lacking that they were secondary growths, and that they did not originate from the nervous tissue itself.

Some of the forms which will be described—the vascular tumors and a sarcoma—can be accepted easily as originating from structures which are normal components of the spinal cord and filum terminale. The same may be true for the neurilemmomas. On the other hand, the origin of tumors such as epidermoids, dermoids, teratomas, and lipomas cannot be explained in this way, hence they must be regarded as arising from heterotopic tissue left behind during the embryonal closing procedure of the spinal cord. That many more of these tumors are found intra-durally and extradurally, extraspinally and subcutaneously, supports the idea that they are the result of congenital malformation. That they are often encountered in combination with spina bifida or spina bifida occulta is additional supporting evidence for this supposition.

We included in this series only those lesions in which there was no evidence of extramedullary continuation of the process. Use of such a standard, we believe, makes it certain that the tumors classified on such a basis originated primarily within the substance of the spinal cord.

Our series is divided into the following groups: vascular tumors (ten cases), sarcoma (one case), epidermoids and dermoids (eight cases), teratoma (two cases), lipomas (six cases), and neurilemmomas (two cases).

VASCULAR TUMORS

Vascular tumors in the spinal cord apparently are rare. So far as we

116

can ascertain, only two major series have been described [Turner and Kernohan[287] (1941) and Wyburn-Mason[310] (1944)]. In addition there are a number of reports of individual cases. Thus the paucity of data about vascular tumors of the spinal cord does not reveal the real incidence of these neoplasms. It also appears that there is no universal agreement regarding the classification of these lesions.

In our series we included only those lesions which were clearly neoplastic; we excluded all the so-called vascular malformations, which are commonly symptomless and which often are incidental findings at necropsy.

The classification employed is that developed by Turner and one of us (Kernohan) in 1941. This system is based on the scheme of Cushing and Bailey[66] (1928), but has been expanded in that it subdivides the neoplasm on the basis of cellularity and cellular activity. In this way were recognized hemangio-endothelioma, hemangioblastoma, and hemangiosarcoma, the first one being the least, and the last one, the most, malignant. The basic structures in these three groups are essentially the same, but the more actively growing tumors possess more cells and exhibit an increased number of mitotic figures.

Histologic Aspects

The most characteristic feature of the hemangio-endothelioma and the hemangioblastoma is the basic network of small vascular channels united with a varying number of larger vessels and sinuses (Fig. 49). The vascular spaces may be either empty or filled with a varying num-

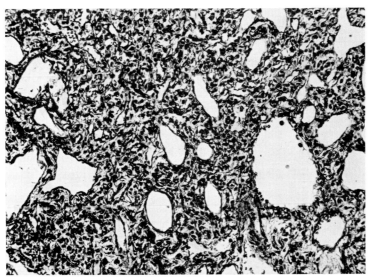

Figure 49. Hemangio-endothelioma, showing vascular channels of varying sizes, lined with endothelial cells. In between are compact masses of endothelial cells (hematoxylin and eosin; × 150).

ber of erythrocytes. As a rule the endothelial cells lining the vessels are fairly uniform and are flattened so that they resemble closely normal endothelial cells. They may, however, contain a fairly large, plump nucleus, which may appear to be slightly pleomorphic. It is not unusual to find some endothelial cells that are swollen and that project into the vascular lumen, sometimes to such an extent that they appear to block the lumen.

It is only rarely that other constituents can be detected as composing the vascular wall, except for a reticulum membrane which is demonstrated when the silver stain is used. Sometimes a varying amount of connective tissue can be seen between the vascular channels. Whether this tissue is an intrinsic part of the wall of the vessel or is the result of degeneration of the tumor remains open to doubt. It is certainly not a constant feature of these tumors.

The spaces between the vessels are filled chiefly by polygonal cells (Fig. 50), which generally have a nucleus of small-to-moderate size. The form of the nucleus may be oval or elongated, but rather often the nuclei vary considerably in form and size. They appear to be somewhat pleomorphic, however, but without a remarkable degree of hyperchromatism in the hemangio-endotheliomas (Fig. 50). Pleomorphism and hyperchromatism increase considerably in the hemangioblastoma and the hemangiosarcoma. The nuclei contain a moderate amount of fine, granular chromatin. Nucleoli are not constant findings, but inclusion-like bodies sometimes can be seen. Mitotic figures usually are absent in the hemangio-endothelioma; a few may be present in the

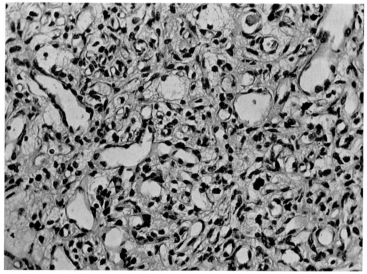

Figure 50. Hemangio-endothelioma, showing slight pleomorphism and irregularity of the tumor cells (hematoxylin and eosin; × 300).

hemangioblastoma, and they are regular features in the hemangio-sarcoma.

The cytoplasm of most of the cells is fairly abundant, but decreases as malignancy increases. For the most part, the cytoplasm appears to be fairly smooth and eosinophilic. Between these cells are cells which have a prominent, foamy or vacuolated cytoplasm (Fig. 51). They usually have a smaller, more rounded nucleus and a well-demarcated cellular membrane. These cells are more abundant in the less malignant tumors. When stained for lipoid, they are seen to contain a Sudan-positive fat. The nature of cells has been interpreted differently, and there is no general agreement whether they are tumor cells or phagocytes. Lindau[176] (1926) thought that they are tumor cells which phagocytize lipoid that is liberated in the process of destruction by the expanding tumor. Tannenberg[282] (1924), however, was of the opinion that these are degenerating tumor cells.

The cellular density in the hemangio-endothelioma is moderate, but in the hemangioblastoma (Fig. 52) and the hemangiosarcoma the density increases considerably as the malignancy increases.

In some of the tumors of our series we found edema, and in a few others a varying amount of connective tissue was noted, sometimes with hyalinization. In an occasional tumor some degree of calcification was present.

Extravasation of erythrocytes and larger hemorrhages are not uncommon. The presence of cells loaded with coarse, brown, iron-containing pigment indicates the occurrence of previous hemorrhages.

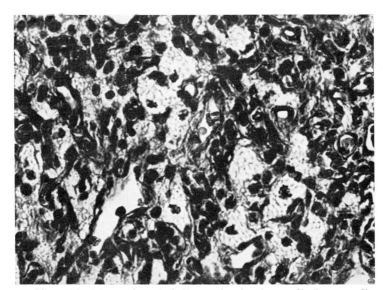

Figure 51. Hemangio-endothelioma, showing foam cells (hematoxylin and eosin; × 400).

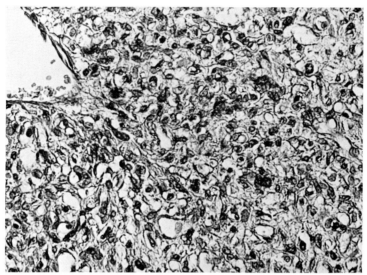

Figure 52. Hemangioblastoma, showing increased nuclear density, irregularity and pleomorphism (hematoxylin and eosin; × 350).

When a reticulum stain is used, an extensive reticulum network (Fig. 53) can be detected which shows many ringlike structures.

Clinical Aspects

Our series of vascular tumors consisted of 10 lesions, five of which were judged to be hemangio-endotheliomas and the remaining five, hemangioblastomas. We did not have an example of hemangiosarcoma.

Seven of the 10 patients were males, and three were females. The average age of patients who had hemangio-endotheliomas was 44 years and 7 months; that of the patients who had hemangioblastomas was 27 years. In the first group, the youngest patient was 30 years old, and the oldest was 51. In the second group, however, the oldest person was 32 years old, and the youngest was 13. It would appear from this that the more malignant tumors develop among persons in a lower age group.

The preoperative duration of symptoms was not significantly different in either group. In the case of hemangio-endotheliomas it was 38 months, and as applicable to hemangioblastomas it was 34 months. In each of both groups we had one instance in which the tumor was found incidentally at necropsy.

The average postoperative survival time among patients who had hemangio-endotheliomas was 99 months. Two patients, however, died of an unrelated disease process: one died of a heart attack or a stroke $8\frac{1}{4}$ years after total removal of such a tumor from the filum terminale, and the other died of carcinoma of the colon 19 years after biopsy and irradiation of a neoplasm in the midthoracic area.

Among patients who had hemangioblastomas, two died postoperatively: one died of a stroke 26 years after total removal, followed by irradiation, of a neoplasm in the midthoracic area, and the other was alive 6 years after biopsy and irradiation for a neoplasm situated in the cervicothoracic area.

The location of the lesions was as follows: two in the cervical area, two in the cervicothoracic area, five in the thoracic area, and one in the filum terminale.

The clinical symptoms were not dissimilar to those caused by gliomas. Pain was the first symptom in six of the eight cases. In one patient a motor, and in another a sensory, disturbance was the first indication of a tumor of the spinal cord.

Five patients were found to have additional symptoms at the time of their physical examination. Results of physical and neurologic examination of two of the remaining patients were negative; one of them had only motor and reflex changes.

In four patients lumbar puncture revealed a complete block when jugular compression was applied. The protein content of the cerebrospinal fluid was increased in the five cases in which it was estimated, the average content being 322 mg. per 100 cc. The lowest protein value was 60 mg. per 100 cc., and the highest, 4000 mg. per 100 cc.

Results of roentgen-ray examination of the spinal column were positive in one patient, and a myelogram made with Pantopaque was diagnostic in the two cases in which myelograms were made.

Four patients died at the Mayo Clinic and thus came to necropsy In

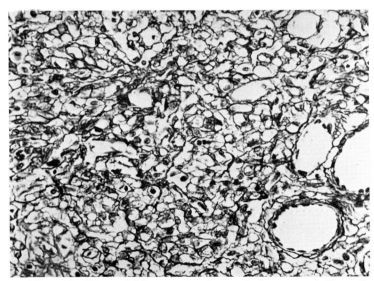

Figure 53. Hemangioblastoma, showing a reticulum network (Gomori's reticulum stain and cresyl violet; × 350).

three of them, additional findings were made, such as angioma in the cerebellum and eyes, cysts in the pancreas, lungs, and kidneys, and carcinoma (hypernephroma) of the kidneys which justified the diagnosis of Lindau-von Hippel disease. In all these patients syringomyelia also was found. Additional information about these cases may be found in Chapter IV, "Vascular Tumors" (cases 38, 39, 40, and 41), p. 174. In none of the remaining six cases did we have clinical evidence to support the diagnosis of Lindau-von Hippel disease, and in these cases the lesions most probably represent solitary vascular tumors without any relationship to the entity of Lindau-von Hippel disease.

SARCOMA

We are unaware of any description in the literature of a primary sarcoma of the spinal cord or filum terminale. Primary sarcoma of the brain is a recognized entity, and according to Uihlein and one of us (Kernohan)[149] it constitutes about 3 per cent of primary intracranial neoplasms.

Report of a Case of Fibrosarcoma of the Filum Terminale

Case 10

A 40-year-old man complained in August, 1959, of pain in the groin, which soon had been followed by weakness in the left leg. In 1958 a hypernephroma had required removal of the left kidney. When he was seen at the Mayo Clinic in October, 1959, sensory disturbance was graded −1, and paralysis of the left leg was graded −2. Reflexes in the same leg were diminished. The protein content of the cerebrospinal fluid was found to be 6000 mg. per 100 cc., with 39 cells per cubic millimeter. Results of roentgenologic examination of the spinal column were negative, but a myelogram made with Pantopaque revealed complete block at the level of the fourth lumbar vertebra. Laminectomy was done from the second to the fourth lumbar vertebrae, and a soft, mushy tumor, 9 cm. long, originating from the filum terminale, was removed. The operation was followed by a course of roentgen-ray therapy.

The patient returned again in February, 1960, at which time he had paraplegia of both legs and difficulties with sphincteric control of the bowel and bladder. A myelogram made with Pantopaque revealed complete block of the cerebrospinal fluid in the lumbar area. Cordectomy, which extended from the level of the tenth thoracic vertebra downward, had to be performed.

The last report received concerning this patient indicated that he was suffering from much pain and that he was moribund.

Histologic examination showed the tumor to be very cellular (Fig. 54). The nuclei were markedly pleomorphic, and varied from spindle-shaped and oval to polygonal. Only an occasional giant nucleus and multinucleated cell were seen. The chromatin content of the nuclei was moderate, and sometimes the chromatin appeared to be finely granular. Many nuclei, however, appeared to be vesicular, with a prominent nuclear membrane. Hyperchromatism was not pronounced. There were many mitotic figures; some were of an abnormal form. Nucleoli were usually absent.

The cellular cytoplasm was scanty and ill-defined. Some cells were recognizable;

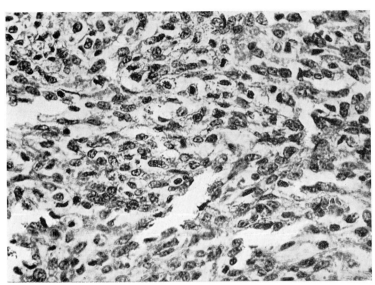

Figure 54. Fibrosarcoma in case 10: marked pleomorphism and hyperchromatism, with several mitotic figures (hematoxylin and eosin; × 350).

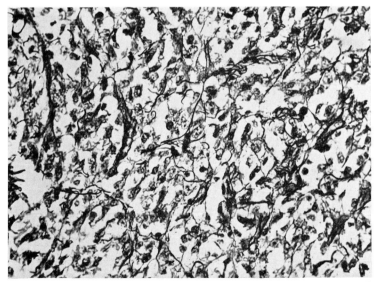

Figure 55. Fibrosarcoma in case 10: irregular reticulum network (Gomori's reticulum stain and cresyl violet; × 350).

when this was true they had an elongated, spindle-shaped form. There were many clear intercellular spaces.

There was some tendency for the cells to be arranged in huge, wavering bundles, but this feature was the only characteristic arrangement that could be recognized.

The tumor was moderately vascular; some swelling of the endothelial cells lining the blood vessels was seen, but marked proliferation was not.

Neither Mallory's phosphotungstic acid stain nor Holzer's stain demonstrated any fibrils, but when Gomori's impregnation technic for reticulum was used, many reticulin fibers were detected, which formed an irregular network (Fig. 55).

Our final diagnosis was highly malignant fibrosarcoma, grade 4.

In the sections of the tissue removed at the second operation no normal tissue of the spinal cord could be recognized at the upper level of the tumor, except for some fibers of the cauda equina which had been partially infiltrated by the tumor.

EPIDERMOIDS, DERMOIDS, AND TERATOMAS

Tumors in this group are commonly regarded as neoplasms of congenital origin in the sense that they are growing and expanding lesions resulting from congenitally misplaced cells. Bostroem[23] in 1897 wrote that Cruveilhier in about 1830 recognized epidermoid tumors as entities and described them as "tumeurs perlées." He thought that these tumors were the results of a fatty secretion in the subarachnoid space. Müller in 1838, according to the same author, gave the first more detailed gross and histologic description of epidermoid tumors, naming them "cholesteatomas" and noting the resemblance of the "cholesteatoma cells" to cornified epidermal cells.

Rokitansky[238] (1856) and others regarded "cholesteatomas" as congeners of the atheromas, and Von Remak[293] (1854) recognized that the "cholesteatomas" of the brain must be derived from epidermal cells left behind in an early phase of the embryologic development (so-called versprengte Keime). Many more theories have been developed during the following years; one of the most prominent was that the epidermoids are derived from endothelial cells (Thoma and others, according to Bostroem).[23]

Bostroem[23] (1897) himself made a thorough embryologic investigation of the pathogenesis of the epidermoids, dermoids, and lipomas. He proved and extended the idea of Von Remak on the displacement of cutaneous-ectodermal cells during the embryologic development of the central nervous system. The displacement is thought to occur early in the fetal development, probably in the third to fifth weeks; this is the period in which the neural groove develops and closes to form the medullary tube, and in which the primitive ectoderm differentiates into cutaneous and neural ectoderm. During this stage it is thought that cutaneous elements can become trapped within or near the newly formed neural tube, and thus can become the basis of an intraspinal or intra-medullary epidermoid or dermoid tumor. It is also thought that when this type of inclusion occurs at an early phase, the cells should be still multipotent, so that teratomas and dermoids will develop. On the other hand, it is postulated, when the inclusion process occurs at a later phase at which the included cells have lost much of their potentiality, an epidermoid will result.

Holmdahl[124] (1933) presented another opinion as to the development of the spinal cord. He suggested that the caudal part of the neural tube develops directly from an undifferentiated cell mass which does not belong to any particular germ layer. The proximal part of the spinal cord is thought to be formed in the way indicated by Bostroem.

List[177] (1941) found this theory to be acceptable. In his opinion it offered an acceptable explanation of the relative frequency of occur-rence of dermoid and other types of embryonic tumors (teratomas) in the lumbosacral area of the spinal cord, ". . . since one has only to as-sume that disorderly differentiation of the primitive matrix causes these tumors."

In the same study List noted that epidermoid tumors occur in a fairly regular distribution over the thoracic and lumbosacral regions of the spinal cord, whereas the dermoid tumors show a definite predilection for the lumbosacral cord.

The explanations as given above are not generally accepted. Holm-dahl's hypothesis was vigorously attacked by Pasteels[210] (1953-1954), who demonstrated that under experimental conditions ectoblastic cells are able to produce heterotopic tissues. Locoge[178] (1958) found the notion unacceptable that ectoblastic cells ("cellules épiblastiques") included in a mass of neuro-ectoblastic cells ("cellules neuro-ectoblastiques") will develop into an epithelial derivant, and he believed that the basis of these congenital tumors is an embryonic deviation, a modification of the potentialities of the young embryonal cells.

According to Furtado and Marques[99] (1951), the present-day concept of the genesis of teratomas is that during embryogenesis a few cells escape the regulating influence of the "primary organizers," grow in accordance with their own intrinsic tendencies, and continue to grow in a complex pluripotential way without any architectural design.

Included in this particular group of congenital tumors is a type of tumor which commonly is regarded as an enterogenous cyst, but which occasionally is described as a "teratoma" or a "teratoid." It is a cystic tumor, the walls of which are lined by entodermal derivates. These cysts can be found in several locations; among these are the intraspinal and intramedullary [Knight-Griffiths-Williams[156] (1954–1955); Rhaney-Bar-clay[226] (1959)].

This rare and extraordinary condition was studied by several investi-gators. Feller and Sternberg[88] (1929) collected 28 cases from the literature and added three of their own, in which there was a gross malformation involving the alimentary canal and the central nervous system. All that these cases had in common was a cleft in the vertebral bodies through which a relationship of the gut and spinal cord became established. In the extreme form the gut simply opened on the back through a cleft in the medullary plate. In the less extreme forms there was a strand or alimentary diverticulum extending to an intact spinal cord. These authors suggested that there might be, at some period of development, a connection between the central nervous system and the alimentary canal, and that a primitive cell rest persisted in the midline, causing a cleft in the notochord. This in turn caused the vertebral anlage to be laid down in two independent halves.

Saunders[248] (1943) felt that an ento-ectodermal adhesion, rather than a primitive cell rest, was the cause for this condition.

Rhaney and Barclay[226] (1959) concluded, from a study of their three cases, that these defects probably result from abnormal separation of the germ layers during embryonic development, and they supported the view that some cysts and diverticula of the alimentary canal and associated vertebral defects are caused by splitting of the notochordal rod, with the exertion of traction between the entodermal tube and the neuro-ectoderm.

It can be concluded from this short and incomplete historical review that the problems concerning the genesis of these congenital tumors are still matters for debate and confusion.

Moreover, it appears to be difficult to form an opinion as to the frequency of occurrence of these tumors, especially since they are uncommon in the intramedullary portion of the spinal cord. A fair number of reports of individual cases have been reported [French-Peyton[98] (1942); Lemmen-Wilson[167] (1951); Verbiest[289] (1939); King[152] (1957); Brizzi[30] (1955); Tinsley-McCoy[286] (1951); Teng-Gordon[285] (1958); Bielschowsky-Unger[21] (1920); and others], but these do not provide a correct impression of the frequency of occurrence of the lesions.

Bradford[26] (1938) concluded, on the basis of study of the literature, that about a third of the reported dermoid and epidermoid tumors of the spinal cord were intramedullary. Leavens, Love, and two of us (MacCarty and Kernohan)[188] in 1959 reported eight intraspinal epidermoid and dermoid tumors among 77 epidermoid tumors of the central nervous system. The location of four of these was intramedullary. Ingraham and Bailey[130] (1946) found 15 teratomas and teratoid tumors among 231 neoplasms of the central nervous system in children. Seven of these were intraspinal; they represented 18 per cent of all the intraspinal tumors. Furtado and Marques[99] (1951) were able to collect from the literature only 10 instances of teratomas in adult persons.

In our material we found 10 lesions which belong to this group of

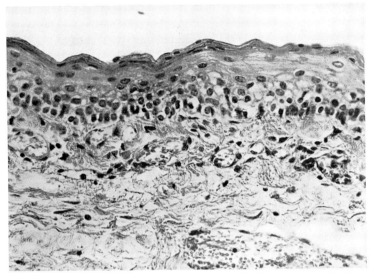

Figure 56. Epidermoid tumor, showing cornified squamous epithelium lining the wall of the cyst (hematoxylin and eosin; × 300).

congenital tumors. Four of these were epidermoid tumors, four were dermoid tumors, and two were classified as teratomas.

Epidermoid Tumors

Epidermoid tumors are cystic lesions; histologically the wall of such a lesion is composed of squamous epithelium (Fig. 56), with intracellular bridges, keratohyalin granules, and cornified cells on the inner surface. These cornified cells become desquamated and form the contents of the cysts. On the outer side of the epithelium is a varying amount of connective tissue, which again may be surrounded by gliosis of the bordering tissue of the spinal cord.

Clinical Findings.   Two of the four patients who had epidermoid tumors were men. The average age of these patients was 45 years and 6 months. The oldest patient was 61 years old, and the youngest was 32 years old. All the tumors were located in the conus medullaris, but two of them had grown beyond that site and had extended along the filum terminale.

The average preoperative duration of the symptoms of these four patients was 12½ years. The shortest duration of symptoms was 8, and the longest, 17 years. One patient had been operated upon before he came to the Mayo Clinic, 6 years after the onset of symptoms.

The first symptom appeared to be variable: in two patients it was pain in the back, in one patient it was dysfunction of the sphincter of the bladder, and in the fourth it was weakness of the legs.

When seen at the Mayo Clinic all four patients exhibited a sensory disturbance in the legs; three had, in addition, saddle anesthesia. Muscular weakness of the legs was found in three patients. All four patients had disturbances of the anal and vesical sphincters. Three had diminished reflexes in the legs, but in one these reflexes were exaggerated.

The average content of protein in the cerebrospinal fluid of three patients was 155 mg. per 100 cc.; the highest content found was 400 mg., and the lowest was 20 mg. Roentgenologic examination of the spinal column showed erosion of the pedicles in three cases, and a myelogram made with Pantopaque revealed partial or total obstruction of the cerebrospinal fluid in the two cases in which this procedure was performed.

All four patients were still alive at the time of this study. The average survival time (computed on the basis of three patients) was 13 years; the longest survival was 20 years. The fourth patient was operated upon recently. This operation was the second he had undergone; it was performed 4 years after the first, which had been carried out elsewhere. One patient was partially, and one was totally, disabled. About the fourth patient we know only that she was alive and had given birth to two children at the time this study was completed.

Dermoid Tumors

Grossly and histologically, the dermoid tumors also are cystic. They are composed of squamous epithelium which cornifies. In addition, they contain skin appendages, such as hair and hair follicles, and sebaceous and sweat glands in the connective tissue below the epithelium. The cysts are filled with the products of these structures, meaning cornified squamous epithelium, hairs, and sebum.

Clinical Findings. We had four examples of dermoid tumors of the intramedullary portion of the spinal cord. The average age of the patients was 31½ years; the oldest was 40 years old, and the youngest was 21 years old. As was true of the epidermoid tumors, all tumors in this group were found in the conus medullaris.

The preoperative duration of symptoms of two patients was 10 years; the third had had symptoms for 2 years; and the fourth had experienced symptoms for only 4 months.

The first symptom related to the presence of this tumor seemed to be variable: it was reported as weakness in the leg or pain in the calf or sacral pain or dysfunction of the bladder and bowel.

When first seen at the Mayo Clinic, three patients had perianal sensory disturbance. One of the three patients had, in addition, a sensory disturbance in the legs, and the fourth patient had a disturbance of pain and temperature sensation in one leg. Three patients were found to have weakness in the legs. Reflex disturbances were present in all four of the patients.

The protein content of the cerebrospinal fluid was markedly elevated (440 mg. per 100 cc.) in one patient and was approximately normal in the remaining three. Roentgenologic examination of the spinal column revealed spondylolisthesis in one patient. A myelogram made with Pantopaque was diagnostic of an intraspinal lesion in all four of the patients.

The length of postoperative survival is known in three cases. One patient underwent re-operation in 1959 for adhesive arachnoiditis, 13 years after the first operation. The second patient was operated upon again in 1960, 8 years after the first procedure, and a recurrent intramedullary tumor was removed from the conus medullaris. The third patient was reported to be doing well 18 years after operation. The fourth patient died, but no further details are known to us.

Teratomas

The definition of a teratoma is still not settled. The description found in the older literature defines a teratoma as a tumor composed of tissues which are derived from all three of the germ layers. Willis[302] (1948) defined a teratoma as a true tumor composed of multiple tissues foreign to the part in which it arises.

We found two examples of teratomas in our series. One was found incidentally at necropsy and is described fully in Chapter IV (case 42).

In the second case a man of 20 years had been suffering from pain in the upper part of the gluteal region for 3 months when he came to the Mayo Clinic in 1951. At examination minimal weakness of the right leg and slight exaggeration of the reflexes in both legs were noted. The protein content of the cerebrospinal fluid was 40 mg. per 100 cc., and there was a complete block of the cerebrospinal fluid, confirmed by a myelogram made with Pantopaque. Roentgenologic examination of the spinal column showed narrowing of the interspace at the third lumbar vertebra. At laminectomy a tumor 5 cm. long was removed. It had originated from the conus medullaris and the filum terminale. The patient reported in 1960, 9 years postoperatively, that he was in good health, but that he noticed some degree of weakness and sensory disturbances in the buttocks and legs.

Histologically, the tumor was found to be composed of cysts lined partially by high cylindric cells which formed finger-like projections into the lumen and partially by ciliated columnar epithelium (Fig. 57). In the surrounding connective tissue were a number of mucous glands which resembled bronchial mucous glands. Some of these were somewhat similar to salivary glands. We also detected areas containing mature fat tissue. In the material that was available there was no evidence of ectodermal derivants such as squamous epithelium, hair, or sebaceous or sweat glands.

In our opinion this tumor represented a teratoma rather than an enterogenous cyst, although most of the structure of the lesion appeared to be of entodermal origin.

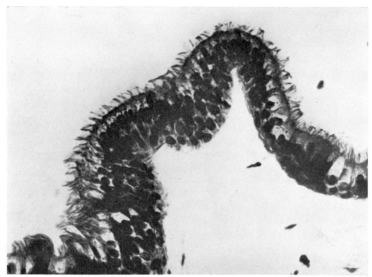

Figure 57.   Teratoma, showing ciliated epithelium as partial lining of a cyst (hematoxylin and eosin; × 400).

LIPOMAS

Intraspinal lipomas are uncommon. Ehni and Love[75] (1945) collected 25 cases from the literature and added four cases from Mayo Clinic material. Johnson[136] (1950) added another seven cases from the literature and one case of his own. Since then, several more reports of individual cases have been added to the literature [Wycis[311] (1953); Crosby-Wagner-Nichols[65] (1953); Slade-Vinas[267] (1956); Nuyts-Hoffman-Haene[203] (1960)].

Fat tissue, abundant in the extradural space, is rarely present in intradural or intramedullary locations. The leptomeninges themselves occasionally contain small amounts of adult fat tissue [Virchow, according to Sperling and Alpers[268] (1936)].

The several theories concerning the development of intradural lipomas were reviewed extensively by Sperling and Alpers[268] (1936) and by Ehni and Love[75] (1945). It is clear, however, that none of them is generally accepted.

Sperling and Alpers (1936) grouped the existing theories into four main categories.

1. The lipoma is hyperplastic growth from normal fat present in the pia mater [Virchow[292] (1864–1865)].

2. Lipomatous tissue is a direct transformation from connective tissue (Pugliese;[218] Naciarone[200]).

3. The lipoma results from displacement or inclusion of embryonal

cells during the formation of the central nervous system from the neural tube [Bostroem[23] (1897); Ernst[86] (1905); Stookey[272] (1927)].

4. Lipomas are aberrant growths related to the development of the primitive layers of the meninges, and they have an embryonic mesenchymal origin (Verga[290]).

To these theories can be added the view of Scherer[253] (1935–1936), who believed that lipomas can develop from the mesenchyma of the local vascular connective tissue.

Ehni and Love[75] (1945) wrote: "Pial lipoma probably arises because of local failure of normal control over formation of fat from the normally present pericapillary mesenchymal cells. In these cells, which have fat-forming potentialities, a panniculus adiposus of the pia proceeds to develop. Whether this is neoplastic or is a 'malformation,' or whether there is any difference between the two, is an open question."

There could be doubt whether lipomas of this type should be included in this study, since it is believed by many investigators that the lesions originate from the pial structures and simply infiltrate the medulla spinalis, being separated from the substance of the spinal cord by a connective tissue membrane of pial origin. We judged it to be justifiable to include lipomas in our study, however, since the symptoms they cause are indistinguishable from those produced by other intramedullary tumors. Moreover, when this type of lipoma is present the surgeon is faced with a lesion on the inner side of the pial membrane, a lesion which is completely adherent to, and indented in, the substance of the spinal cord.

We found six cases in which the surgeon had reported a lipoma to be situated in a completely intramedullary position.

Histologic Aspects

The microscopic picture of the lipomas is extremely simple. It is not distinguishable from the microscopic picture of normal adult fat tissue. A section is seen to be composed of huge cells which are optically clear when stained with hematoxylin and eosin (Fig. 58), but which are brilliant red when treated with Sudan IV stain. The cells are pressed together and are of various shapes, but as a rule are polygonal. Sharp, thin, cellular membranes are seen. The nuclei are relatively small, and are compressed against the cellular membrane. The histologic diagnosis of lipoma must be supported by gross and clinical evidence, since there are no histologic diagnostic criteria which separate the lipoma from mature fat tissue.

Between the fat cells small rims of connective tissue and blood vessels can be found.

Clinical Aspects

Of our six patients who had lipomas, only one was a female. The ages varied greatly, and we were unable to confirm the predominance, ac-

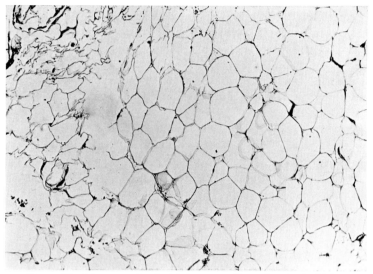

Figure 58. Lipoma stained with hematoxylin and eosin (× 100).

cording to age groups, reported by Ehni and Love. The patients were, respectively, 8, 19, 22, 45, 56, and 61 years of age. The preoperative duration of symptoms averaged 11 years and 8 months. The shortest preoperative duration of symptoms was 3 years and 9 months, and the longest was 31 years. Pain was the first symptom of four patients; the fifth reported an impression of deadness in his toes. The initial symptom of the sixth patient was difficult to evaluate, since this man also had progressive spastic paraplegia which followed an injury, with a compression fracture of the first lumbar vertebra.

At the time of their first examination all patients were found to have motor disturbances and abnormal reflexes. A sensory disturbance was noted in only four patients.

The protein content of the cerebrospinal fluid averaged 60 mg. per 100 cc. in four patients; in the fifth it was 1000 mg. per 100 cc., but partial block of the cerebrospinal fluid was found in this man.

Roentgenologic examination of the spinal column revealed an anomaly of the vertebrae in two patients (spina bifida occulta). A myelogram made with Pantopaque was diagnostic of an intraspinal tumor in four patients and was indeterminate in one.

In the surgical reports the tumor was described as being in an intramedullary position. In two cases it was present in the cervical segment of the spinal cord, in one case in the thoracic segment of the cord, and in three cases in the conus medullaris. In none of the cases could complete removal be performed.

Four patients answered requests for follow-up information. The fifth patient was known to have been alive in 1958, 15 years after operation.

The average survival time was 12 years; the longest survival period was 33 years, and the shortest was 3 years. All patients, however, appeared to have been partially or totally disabled.

NEURILEMMOMA

Reports in the literature of an intramedullary neurilemmoma are extremely rare. Except for the Mayo Clinic material, so far as we have been able to determine, only three reports of this lesion have been published [Riggs-Clary[230] (1957); Ramamurthi-Anguli-Iyer[221] (1958); Scott-Bentz[261] (1962)]. According to Ramamurthi and associates, a fourth case should be present in the literature, but we have been unable to locate this case.

As was mentioned in relation to extramedullary neurilemmomas (Chapter I), the histogenesis of this type of lesion is still unsettled, but the relationship of neurilemmomas to peripheral nerves is beyond doubt. It is common knowledge that peripheral or sympathetic nerves sometimes can be demonstrated in the substance of the spinal cord, especially in the thoracic (Fig. 59) and lumbar sections of the cord, and then mostly in a perivascular position. One of us [Kernohan[143] (1941)] wrote that these nerves can be the sources of an intramedullary neurilemmoma, and Riggs and Clary[230] (1957) also wrote of such an occurrence. Ramamurthi and associates[221] pointed to a mechanism of inclusion of cells of the

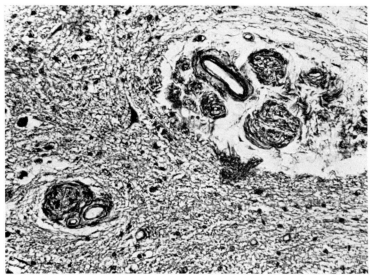

Figure 59. Section from the thoracic segment of the spinal cord, showing the intramedullary nerves in the perivascular space (hematoxylin and eosin; × 200).

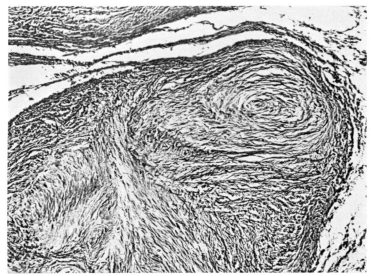

Figure 60. Neurilemmoma, showing wavering bands of cells and palisading (hematoxylin and eosin; × 150).

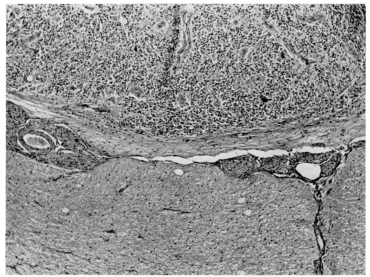

Figure 61. Two small perivascular neurilemmomas situated anteriad to the grade 1 cellular ependymoma in case 19, Chapter IV (hematoxylin and eosin; × 50).

neural crest in the neural tube, similar to the process which is thought to occur in the case of epidermoid and dermoid tumors.

In our records we found one case which has been reported previously [Kernohan (1932[141]) and (1941[143])]. The patient was a boy 12 years old who experienced progressive pain in the arms, followed by loss of strength in the arms and legs during a period of 4 years. At examination loss of sensation in the arms, trunk, and legs and weakness in the upper and lower extremities were found. Reflexes were absent in the arms and were slightly exaggerated in the legs. At operation an intramedullary tumor was removed subtotally from the spinal cord in the fourth to the seventh cervical segments. Follow-up information about this patient was not available.

Histologically (Fig. 60), the tumor had the same structure as that of the extramedullary neurilemmomas (Chapter I).

In one other case (case 19 in Chapter IV) we found three small structures composed of Schwann cells which probably represented neurilemmomas. They were located anteriad to an ependymoma (Fig. 61). These structures were much larger than normal nerves as found in the spinal cord. The histologic character and the size of these lesions caused us to judge that they represented neurilemmomas.

IV

Postmortem Examinations

Postmortem examinations as performed in 33 cases gave us the opportunity to study some details which had remained obscure in surgically removed material. In this way we obtained a better understanding of the extent and location of the tumor and the relationship of the lesion to the normal structures. Such data from necropsy also might assist in a better understanding of the relationship of tumors to syringomyelia.

First we shall present clinical and anatomical descriptions of the cases, grouped according to the type of tumor present. Next we shall offer a discussion concerning several features.

The series we have available includes eight astrocytomas, one spongioblastoma, 13 ependymomas, two oligodendrogliomas, four instances of Von Recklinghausen's disease, four vascular neoplasms, and one teratoma of the spinal cord.

ASTROCYTOMAS

Case 5*

A man 27 years old had noted, since 1946, 3 years before he died, progressive sensory and motor dysfunction in the lower half of the body. At the first operation a tumor of the spinal cord could not be located, but after several courses of roentgen-ray therapy, at operation in 1948 a highly malignant tumor was found in the upper part of the thoracic segment of the cord. Cordectomy was performed. The patient died after having manifested the signs of intracranial involvement.

Necropsy. Bilateral bronchopneumonia, hepatosplenomegaly, caused by hemosiderosis, acute duodenal ulcers, and hypertrophy of the adrenal glands were found.

* The clinical details in this case are given in Chapter II.

136

Gross examination of the brain, cerebellum, and brain stem disclosed no abnormalities. In cross sections, however, several apparently independent tumor masses were found. In the left frontal horn, closely adherent to the anterior tip of the caudate nucleus, was an irregular, red tumor mass, approximately 1 cm. in diameter and soft and mushy.

A second tumor mass was found in the right frontal lobe close to the septum pellucidum. It extended into the lateral ventricle from the tip of the anterior horn posteriorly to the level of the massa intermedia. The lower part of the tumor had pushed through the foramen of Monro and extended down the right wall of the third ventricle to the left of the anterior commissure. It extended posteriad to touch the massa intermedia, where it ended. This tumor was red, glossy on the external surface, and felt nodular to palpation.

The upper half of the fourth ventricle was completely filled with a tumor which appeared to be homogeneous; it was pale pinkish and soft and fleshy. It extended cephalad from the level of the lateral recesses to end at the beginning of the aqueduct of Sylvius, but this passage appeared to be free of tumor.

The cerebellum appeared to be normal except for an indefinite infiltration at a point at which it overlaid the tumor in the roof of the fourth ventricle.

The cervical portion of the spinal cord was not removed, but the first few segments which were obtained were free of tumor.

Histologic Aspects.   The surgical specimen of the spinal cord contained a tumor which extended from the upper part of the thoracic level to the lumbar area. The sacral segment of the cord, the filum terminale, and the cauda equina were free of tumor. In the midthoracic portion of the cord the tumor was most extensive and also most malignant; it was a grade 4 astrocytoma. In some areas the tumor was extremely cellular and pleomorphic, with many giant nuclei and multinucleated cells and fairly marked hyperchromatism. A moderate number of mitotic figures were seen. A certain number of cells could be fairly easily recognized as being, or being derived from, fibrillary astrocytes (Fig. 13). In some places groups of gemistocytic astrocytes were present.

Vascularity was increased, and there was also moderate endothelial proliferation in the walls of the blood vessels. Areas of necrosis were not seen.

At the midthoracic level of the spinal cord the normal anatomic relationships were completely disorganized and unrecognizable; a few nerve cells were found scattered about and the only structure which could be identified was a group of ependymal cells in what had been the central canal.

The tumor extended to the surface of the cord all about the circumference of that structure, but did not proceed beyond that area.

In the upper part of the thoracic segment of the spinal cord, as well as in the lumbar part of the cord, the tumor was less cellular, and was seen to be infiltrating between normal structures, which were still recognizable as such. Infiltration seemed to be the heaviest in the medial area of the dorsal half of the cord, but extended to a lesser degree beyond that area. The grade of malignancy in several areas was lower, and the lesion in those locations was a grade 2 astrocytoma.

In no place was syringomyelia found.

All the tumors in the brain were similar, and all had the characteristics of a grade 4 astrocytoma. The difference between them and the tumor in the spinal cord was that those of the brain contained more and larger giant nuclei and multinucleated cells and more mitotic figures, but no necrosis. The tumor infiltrated diffusely into the neighboring substance of the brain and in many places reached the ventricular surfaces and was seen to extend below a layer of ependymal cells.

Conclusion.   A grade 4 astrocytoma of the spinal cord extended into the thoracic and lumbar segments, and caused symptoms for almost 3 years. In three separate locations of the brain there were also grade 4 astrocytomas which had caused symptoms only during the last part of the patient's life.

There remained the question whether there was any relationship among these four tumors. Did those in the brain represent metastasis from the tumor of the spinal cord or did they develop independently as a consequence of a general tendency toward neoplastic genesis within the nervous system? Because metastatic lesions were not found elsewhere, and especially not in the subarachnoid space, we think that each of these tumors was an independent neoplasm with multiple foci of origin.

Another example of the multifocal development of tumors will be described in the section dealing with Von Recklinghausen's disease.

Case 11

The patient was a 44-year-old woman who, 54 months before her death in 1952, had complained of pain in the interscapular area which was worse at night and extended to the anterior wall of the thorax. She also complained of a transient sense of numbness in the region of the left hip, and some pain which extended down the left leg and was aggravated by bending and stooping movements. Results of physical examinations at this time were negative.

A year later pain extended to an upper abdominal quadrant. Complete studies revealed gallstones. The only neurologic finding was a value for protein in the cerebrospinal fluid of 100 mg. per 100 cc. Cholecystectomy was performed.

The patient remained relatively comfortable for 2 years, but then pain developed in the neck and the left leg and arm, accompanied by weakness of the left leg and shaking in the right hand. She also had headache and vomiting and experienced difficulty in voiding. A neurologic examination, performed elsewhere, is said to have revealed evidence of compression of the spinal cord at the level demarcated by the first and second thoracic vertebrae. The content of protein in the cerebrospinal fluid was 840 mg. per 100 cc., and there were 54 lymphocytes per cubic millimeter of fluid. Myelographic studies showed a subarachnoid obstruction at the level of the third thoracic vertebra. Laminectomy, extending from the seventh cervical to the fifth thoracic vertebrae,* was done. Dense adhesions were seen between the dura and ligamentum and the dorsal aspect of the cord at the level of the third thoracic vertebra. The cord did not pulsate, but seemed normal in consistency. Numerous dilated vascular channels had developed over the dorsal aspect of the spinal cord, but incision of the cord did not give evidence of tumor or cystic degeneration.

The patient's pain appeared to have been significantly relieved by the operative procedure, but otherwise there was no essential change in her neurologic condition.

Eight months before the death of this patient the left leg became numb and flexion contracture developed; she complained again of severe pain in the head and neck. The impression that the patient had an intramedullary tumor of the spinal cord persisted; deep roentgen-ray therapy was administered. It produced considerable relief of symptoms for about 4 months. Another myelogram disclosed block of the cerebrospinal fluid at the cervicothoracic level. Roentgen-ray therapy was repeated.

The patient was admitted to a hospital in Rochester, Minnesota, 5 days before death, complaining chiefly of pain in the neck and head. Neurologic examination demonstrated spastic paralysis of both legs, anesthesia from about the nipple downward which was gradually extending distally; reflexes in the legs were

* The exposure from the third cervical to the tenth thoracic vertebrae, described in the appendix, was obtained at necropsy.

absent, as were the abdominal reflexes. Bilateral papilledema of 6 diopters was noted. The cranial nerves were unremarkable. Results of roentgenologic examination of the spinal column and skull were negative. The patient's condition rapidly deteriorated, and she died on the fifth day after admission, death being caused by respiratory failure.

Necropsy. Acute pyelonephritis of the right kidney, with hemorrhagic cystitis, was found.

The brain was normal except for a small amount of old blood pigment in the subarachnoid space over the inferior surface of the cerebellum. The entire spinal cord was two to three times normal size, and was brown and mushy. The entire cervical portion of the cord was cystic. The diameter of the cyst was 1 cm., and the cyst was lined by brown mucoid material. Discoloration and abnormality in consistency extended into the lower portion of the medulla. The cord was hemorrhagic and necrotic down to the lumbar region. A mucoid tumor was found to involve the cauda equina, matting the roots together. There was a moderate amount of old, thick, dark blood in the subarachnoid space around the spinal cord.

Histologic Aspects. Histologic examination showed that the components of the tumor extended continuously from the second cervical to the first lumbar roots. The tumor was essentially a moderately edematous grade 1 astrocytoma, located mainly in the central area of the spinal cord just dorsal to the central canal. At the level of the third thoracic vertebra the tumor tissue reached the dorsal surface of the cord. Laterally, the tumor extended in the mid-dorsal area beyond the dorsal and ventral horns; in only a few places in this area could remaining ganglion cells be found. There they appeared to be embedded in the tumor tissue. In many places the periphery of the tumor was irregular and indistinct, consisting mostly of pre-existing spinal-cord tissue invaded by tumor cells. In a number of sections it was remarkable that there was a marked increase of oligodendrocytes around the tumor and in the zone invaded by tumor.

Several areas in the tumor contained cell groups which were more pleomorphic and anaplastic, and which contained occasional mitotic figures. There were also a few binucleated cells but no bizarre or giant nuclei. The cellular density of these areas also was increased. These more malignant-appearing areas were located chiefly in the center of the tumor and were surrounded by zones of tissue of grade 1 malignancy. Slight-to-moderate increased vascularity was detected, but many vessels exhibited remarkable endothelial swelling without, however, too-prominent proliferation.

Inside the tumor we found extensive, fresh hemorrhage which extended from the lower cervical level through the whole tumor and into the lumbar and sacral segments of the cord. In addition, in many places, cells were present which contained coarse brown granules indicating old hemorrhage.

The upper thoracic portion of the cord appeared to be infarcted. It was invaded by erythrocytes.

Microscopically, the cyst in the cervical portion of the cord was a syringomyelic cavity the wall of which was composed chiefly of dense glial tissue (Fig. 62), abundant in neuroglial fibrils (Fig. 63), and containing innumerable Rosenthal fibers. In the syringomyelic wall several groups of cells were found which were full of brown iron pigment. The upper segments of the cord had the appearance of having been unfolded, and the dorsal horns were found at the lateral edges of the cord. The dorsal wall of the cavity consisted only of glial tissue. In two lateral areas in the upper part of the cervical segment of the cord the dense glial tissue had been partially or totally replaced by a small group of tumor cells. At the level of the fourth cervical vertebra the cord appeared to be "closed," and contained a large cavity which, on one dorsolateral side, was lined by the tumor tissue. Gang-

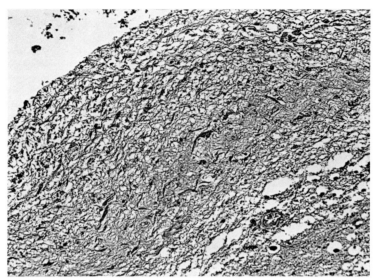

Figure 62. Wall of syringomyelic cavity in case 11, Chapter IV, showing moderately dense glial network with several Rosenthal fibers (hematoxylin and eosin; × 125).

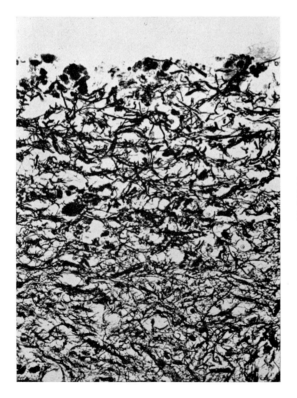

Figure 63. Same case as in Figure 62: wall of syringomyelic cavity, showing network of glial fibrils and some Rosenthal fibers (Holzer stain; × 300).

lion cells of the dorsal and ventral horns were present, but appeared to be compressed and partly degenerated. Ventral to the syrinx a group of ependymal cells was found; these cells appeared to be disorganized and did not form a canal.

At the cervicothoracic juncture the tumor mass had expanded itself, and there was no longer any indication of a pre-existing syringomyelic cavity. From this site the tumor extended as one mass downward to the low thoracic area.

In the central portion of the lumbar segment of the cord extensive hemorrhage was seen. At this point there was no indication of tumor tissue or of a pre-existing cavity. There was, however, an area in which moderate gliosis was seen and in which many Rosenthal fibers were recognized. The normal structures in this segment of the cord were well preserved, but calcification of the walls of vessels was remarkable. Several cell groups were loaded with iron pigment, indicating old hemorrhage. The nerve roots of the cauda equina were embedded in a tumor mass which had all the characteristics of a grade 1 astrocytoma. There was no apparent invasion of the roots by the tumor.

Conclusion. A 44-year-old woman had exhibited for 4½ years symptoms referable to a disease of the spinal cord, the nature of which, even at operation, was not clear. At necropsy a large syringomyelic cavity was found in the cervical segment of the cord, and a predominantly grade 1 astrocytoma, extending through the total length of the thoracic segment of the cord and extending up into the syringomyelic wall was disclosed. Extensive hemorrhage had occurred in the tumor, and focal, partially hemorrhagic, necrosis had taken place in the upper part of the thoracic segment of the cord. The cauda equina was embedded in the same type of tumor, which very likely was metastatic.

Case 12

At the age of 6 months (in 1946) a male child had been noted to be constipated. At about the same time the mother also saw that the infant stiffened his legs when she changed his diapers.

When the child was seen at the Mayo Clinic muscle strength could not be detected below the level of the shoulder girdle, and there were no spontaneous movements in the legs. Reflexes in the legs were brisk; Babinski's sign was elicited bilaterally. No specific diagnosis could be made at this time, and no treatment was administered.

Three months later the condition appeared to be essentially unchanged, although, lately, a few spontaneous movements in the legs and a reaction to painful stimuli were noted. The protein content of the cerebrospinal fluid was 750 mg. per 100 cc., with only 1 lymphocyte per cubic millimeter. Roentgenograms of the thorax and spinal column disclosed nothing of significance. A ventriculogram was made, and this revealed secondary dilatation of the ventricular system. A lesion of the spinal cord was now suspected.

The patient returned at the age of 16 months, a victim of pneumonia in the upper lobe of the right lung. Muscles of the legs were still weak. Function of the arms apparently was normal. The child died 2 days after admission.

Necropsy. The immediate cause of death was determined as bilateral bronchopneumonia.

The upper part of the thoracic cavity contained a lobulated mass of soft, yellow-pinkish-white tissue which had a fairly distinct capsule. This mass, 8 by 5 cm., was seen to be overlying the bodies of the first three thoracic vertebrae. Cross sections of the vertebral bodies revealed that this tissue had extended into the widened vertebral canal through the lateral foramina, where it had compressed the dura and the cord to the size of a thin ribbon over the distance of these three vertebrae. The dura was not penetrated by this tissue.

Histologic Aspects.   Histologically, the tumor mass was a fibromyxosarcoma. In none of the sections could invasion of the dura be observed, and the intradural space was free of tumor.

Surprisingly, in the spinal cord, at the level of the second and third thoracic vertebrae, we found a grade 1 astrocytoma, 4 by 6 mm. This tumor was located in the midline of the dorsal half of the cord, and it had pushed both dorsal horns lateroventrally and was completely surrounded by normal spinal-cord tissue. The central canal was easily recognizable. It was located slightly to one side and anteriad to the tumor.

In several places the periphery of the tumor was fairly sharply demarcated (Fig. 64), but in other areas the surrounding portion of the cord had been invaded. In the center of the tumor a few calcium deposits were found.

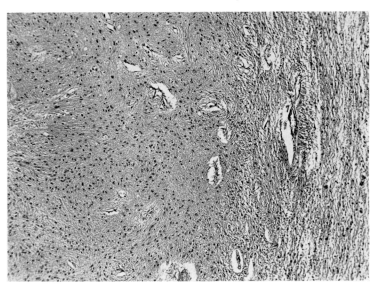

Figure 64. Grade 1 astrocytoma in case 12 in Chapter IV. There is a fairly sharp demarcation at the line of juncture with normal tissue (hematoxylin and eosin; × 100).

Conclusion.   This 16-month-old boy, suffering for about 10 months from disease of the spinal cord, had at approximately the same vertebral level an extradural and extraspinal fibromyxosarcoma and an intramedullary grade 1 astrocytoma. It appears, however, unlikely that the presence of the astrocytoma could explain all the clinical findings.

Case 13

A woman 48 years old was seen at the Mayo Clinic in 1944, 3 weeks before her death, complaining chiefly of increasing pain in the neck of 10 months' duration, aggravated by coughing. Numbness and weakness of the arms and legs had been present for 6 months. Shortly before she was seen at the Mayo Clinic difficulty with the bladder had developed. Three years previously the patient had undergone removal of a carcinoma of the breast.

Definite diminution of sensation to touch was found, and sensation of pain and temperature was equally diminished on both sides in the upper half of the body, but was more marked on the right side in the lower half of the body. The upper level was at or near the fifth cervical segment. Weakness was equal in both arms; Babinski's sign was elicited on the right. The cerebrospinal fluid was slightly xanthochromic; the protein content was 1000 mg. per 100 cc.

Bilateral laminectomy was done; it extended from the fourth to the seventh cervical vertebrae.* The spinal cord felt very firm; after incision a blue granular material was seen. A specimen was taken for biopsy, and the dura was left open.

Postoperatively the course of the patient declined slowly. Weakness of the arms gradually increased, as did temperature and dyspnea. Finally, coma supervened and death occurred 14 days after the operation.

Necropsy. The brain was edematous; petechial hemorrhages had developed in the left temporal lobe.

A tumor mass 6 cm. long and 2 cm. in diameter was found in the substance of the cervical part of the cord. The tumor was soft and yellow-white.

Histologic Aspects. Nearly the entire cross section of the spinal cord was involved by the tumor: only both dorsolateral areas were free from the neoplastic lesion. In both ventral and dorsal horns the ganglion cells still could be detected, but the number of them had decreased. In many other fields fiber tracts were recognized, but they were separated and split by the invading tumor cells.

In most areas the tumor was a moderately cellular, fibrillary astrocytoma with slight pleomorphism—a grade 1 astrocytoma. In one area, however, cellularity and pleomorphism were increased, and some small giant nuclei and a few mitoses were present. This latter area appeared to be completely embedded in the less malignant tumor, and the tissue concerned was diagnosed as a grade 3 astrocytoma. Vascularity was moderate in most of the tumor, but was more pronounced in the area of greater malignancy.

In several areas of the tumor groups of gemistocytic astrocytes were found (Fig. 6). In the vicinity of the site from which a specimen had been taken for biopsy some degree of degeneration and gitter cells were seen. Otherwise, necrosis had not developed in the tumor.

Syringomyelia was not found.

Conclusion. A 48-year-old woman who had been suffering pain in the neck for 10 months, and progressive quadriparesis, was found to have an astrocytoma of moderate size almost completely replacing the cervical segment of the spinal cord. Eighty to 90 per cent of the tumor had the appearance of a lesion of grade 1 malignancy, but in one area the malignant factor had increased to that of a fairly active grade 3 astrocytoma. There was no indication of syringomyelia.

Case 14

Eight years before his death in 1916, a man 34 years old noticed gradually increasing weakness of the left leg. Five years after the onset of this difficulty he had been temporarily confined to a wheelchair.

In 1916 he had undergone an operation on the back in which "incision of the cord" had been done. Subsequently, braces were applied.

Rapidly increasing weakness of the right leg started 11 months before death of the patient. At times there was loss of control of the bowel and bladder.

Neurologic examination demonstrated weakness in both legs, more pronounced in the left leg than in the right, with atrophy of the left leg and bilaterally diminished reflexes. From the waist down there was complete absence of sensation for all modalities.

Roentgenologic examination of the spinal column and lumbar puncture produced nothing significant.

Laminectomy was done; it extended from the seventh through the ninth

* Surgical exposure. At necropsy (see appendix) the exposure was at the fifth and
   sixth cervical vertebrae.

thoracic vertebrae.* A soft tumor in the substance of the spinal cord, extending for about 1 inch, was found, and a portion of it was removed. The dura was left open.

Postoperatively, trophic ulcers developed over the sacrum and the patient had much difficulty in control of his bladder and bowels. He died 3 months after the operation. Death was caused by septicemia arising from the trophic ulcers.

Necropsy.   Trophic ulcers were found on both hips, knees, and heels; and a psoas abscess was discovered on the right. Hydropericardium, with chronic myocarditis, and edema of the lungs also were present.

In the spinal cord, extending from the level of the tenth thoracic vertebra to and including part of the cauda equina there was a large jelly-like mass which apparently had replaced the cord. This mass was mottled pink and yellow, very soft in consistency and rich in blood supply.

Histologic Aspects.   In the sections the lower part of the cord appeared to be completely replaced by a moderately cellular, fibrillary astrocytoma of grade 1 malignancy. In most areas the tumor was slightly edematous, and in some areas a few Rosenthal fibers were present.

In the thoracic segment of the cord, above the tumor, extending up to the cervical area, a slitlike cavity (Fig. 65) was found, the wall of which was composed

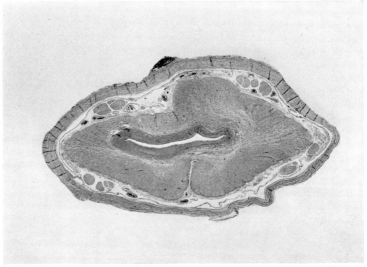

Figure 65.   Syringomyelia in case 14 in Chapter IV (hematoxylin and eosin; × 5).

of dense glial tissue, with relatively few cells and numerous neuroglial fibrils. In this wall many Rosenthal fibers of all shapes and sizes were found, and there also were some iron-containing cells. In the cavity itself a few gitter cells were seen. The cavity was located on one side of the cord, and had pushed the dorsal horn ventrolateral. The dorsal septum of the cord and a persistent central canal had been pushed toward the opposite side, and there was no relationship between the syringomyelia and the central canal.

Conclusion.   A 34-year-old man, who for 8 years had been a victim of weakness of the legs, was found to have had a grade 1 astrocytoma which had completely

* Necropsy (see appendix) showed that the tumor actually extended further downward than this.

replaced the lower part of the thoracic segment and the lumbar segment of the spinal cord, and syringomyelia in the levels above the tumor, extending up to the cervical part of the cord.

Case 15

A man 46 years old in 1947 had experienced episodes of pain in the back, generally initiated after bending or lifting. He would be unable to straighten up, and occasionally he suffered sciatic pain. A myelogram made with Pantopaque revealed a protruded intervertebral disk. Surgical removal of two ruptured intervertebral disks at the lumbosacral level and at the fourth lumbar interspaces was carried out. This relieved him of his difficulty, but 6 months later similar pain arose. He used a belt to relieve the pain.

In 1950 the patient returned complaining of intermittent numbness and tingling in the right foot and leg of about 2 years' duration. He said that sometimes he experienced a sensation such as that imparted by a constricting bandage around the right knee. For a year he had had pain in the right arm, and for a shorter period pain had been present in the shoulder and left hand. The pain was thought to be the result of periarthritis.

The patient was seen again in 1957, 3 weeks before his death. A grade 4 squamous-cell carcinoma was detected in the upper lobe of the left lung. Metastasis had occurred, and migratory thrombophlebitis was present in the right arm and in both legs. He was treated with roentgen ray therapy

The only hint of the presence of a lesion of the spinal cord was that coughing would cause marked pain over the right lower anterior ribs.

The patient died 3 weeks after his admission.

Necropsy. In addition to the bronchogenic carcinoma with multiple metastases, already mentioned, a paraphyseal cyst of the third ventricle of the brain was found between the foramina of Monro. In the spinal cord a syringomyelic cavity was disclosed, and there was an intramedullary astrocytoma in the cervical and upper thoracic portions of the cord.

Histologic Aspects. A slitlike syringomyelic cavity was found extending from the level of the third cervical to that of the fifth thoracic root. The wall of this cavity was composed of fairly dense glial tissue with a low-to-moderate cell content, and an abundance of glial fibrils with several Rosenthal fibers. In one area the cavity was partially lined by a small group of cuboidal ependymal cells which were clearly separated from the central canal, which was located anteriad to the cavity. In the upper levels of the cord the syringomyelic defect was centrally located, but had developed laterally in the lower levels.

In the substance of the cord between the fourth and the sixth cervical vertebrae was a small group of fibrillary astrocytes. At the upper level this group of astrocytes was situated adjacent to, but at the lower level was separated from, the lateral edge of the syringomyelia. This formation was moderately cellular, somewhat edematous, and contained only a few Rosenthal fibrils. Pleomorphism was slightly more pronounced than that in the gliotic tissue of the syringomyelic cavity wall, but there were no giant cells or mitotic figures. This cell group represented a small grade 1 astrocytoma.

Conclusion. This 46-year-old man probably had two instances of difficulty referable to the spinal cord. In the first episode the distress was caused by two ruptured intervertebral disks; in the second one, commencing 7 years before his death, the difficulty probably was caused by syringomyelia which affected the cord from the level of the second cervical to that of the fifth thoracic vertebrae, and by a small astrocytoma of the cord between the fourth and sixth cervical segments.

Case 16

A woman 21 years old had noted in 1922, a year before she was operated upon, pain in the neck and right shoulder which was aggravated by her sitting or lying down. This pain caused sleeplessness at night. It became progressively worse and extended into the right arm and forearm. Three months later numbness and weakness began in the right hand, and later extended into the arm. Ten months after the beginning of this difficulty weakness, numbness, and paresthesia developed in the right leg, and pain and paresthesia were present in the left arm.

A month before the patient came to the Mayo Clinic she experienced headaches and signs of incontinence.

Neurologic examination disclosed weakness of the right side of the body, atrophy of the small muscles of the right hand, and tendon reflexes which were diminished in the arms but were slightly exaggerated in the legs. Babinski's sign was elicited bilaterally, but was more pronounced on the right. Sensation of pain and temperature was slightly impaired, and was more noticeable on the left. Roentgenologic examination produced nothing of significance. The reaction of the Nonne-Apelt procedure on the cerebrospinal fluid was positive; the fluid contained 5 cells per cubic millimeter.

Laminectomy was done at the level of the sixth and seventh cervical vertebrae. The spinal cord was seen to be enlarged to about twice normal size, and it was bulging. An intramedullary glioma was found in the cord at the level in question. Decompression of the spinal cord was done.

In the evening of the same day a high temperature developed; the patient became stuporous and died some hours later of progressive respiratory failure.

Necropsy.   In general, the body and brain were essentially normal. An ovoid swelling was seen in the spinal cord in the level of the fifth to the seventh cervical vertebrae.* Cross-sectioning disclosed a centrally located intramedullary tumor.

Histologic Aspects.   The tumor was found to be sharply delineated. It was 1.9 cm. in largest diameter. It was a moderately cellular, grade 2 astrocytoma with some degree of pleomorphism, but hyperchromatism was not remarkable. The tumor cells were grouped in intermingling bundles of various sizes. With Mallory-phosphotungstic acid stain a moderate number of neuroglial fibrils were seen. The tumor was moderately vascular; there was no endothelial proliferation of the walls of the blood vessels. At the outer borders of the tumor typical neoplastic fibrillary astrocytes were recognized.

The pre-existent tissue of the spinal cord was compressed to a small rim around the tumor. The normal anatomic structures were distorted, but a number of nerve cells of the anterior horns could still be recognized. A central canal in the cord could not be found at the level of the tumor.

In the spinal cord, at a point above the site of the tumor, a small intramedullary hemorrhage was present. Syringomyelia was not found.

Conclusion.   A woman 21 years old who had suffered for a year from the effects of disease of the spinal cord was found to have had a grade 2 astrocytoma which extended from approximately the level of the fifth to that of the seventh cervical vertebrae. Syringomyelia was not present.

Case 17

A girl 14 years old was seen in 1923 with weakness in the legs that had started in the right ankle and 2½ months later had shifted to the left leg. The duration

* The exact location of the lesion (see appendix) later was found to be between the sixth and seventh cervical vertebrae.

of this weakness was 4 months. Ankle clonus was noted in both legs, and the patient complained of mild pain in the left lumbar region on bending the head forward. Some degree of incontinence of urine had been present for 2 months, and constipation was reported.

It was found that the patient had nearly complete paralysis of both legs, and that anesthesia and analgesia extended to the level of the ninth thoracic vertebra. Abdominal reflexes and knee reflexes were absent; the Achilles reflexes were exaggerated. Babinski's sign was elicited bilaterally.

Roentgenograms of the spinal column disclosed nothing of significance.

Exploratory laminectomy was done; it extended from the sixth to the tenth thoracic vertebrae. The spinal cord appeared to be fusiform; it was covered with numerous congested vessels. In the middle portion (the seventh to eighth thoracic vertebrae) a grayish-pink tumor extended through the substance of the cord. It was about 5 cm. long and 2.5 cm. in diameter, and could not be removed.

The patient's condition remained about the same as it had been prior to the operation. Treatments with radium were given. Six months after the operation information was received that the patient had died. Her condition had deteriorated steadily, and the paralysis had extended into both upper extremities. Six weeks before her death pyelonephritis developed, and the patient died in uremic coma.

A part of the spinal cord was sent to us for study.

Histologic Aspects. The tumor was a cellular grade 4 astrocytoma with marked pleomorphism and hyperchromatism and many bizarre giant nuclei and multinucleated cells (Fig. 12) The number of mitotic figures was moderate. In some areas the cellularity and the anaplasia were less and the tumor cells were readily recognizable as astrocytic derivations. Markedly increased vascularity and moderate endothelial proliferation were seen.

In most of the cross sections the complete cord appeared to have been infiltrated, and in most places the tumor extended to the surface. The only remnant of normal structures was an occasional nerve cell in an area in which the grade of malignancy was lower.

Conclusion. In a 14-year-old girl who had been suffering for 10 months from the effects of a tumor of the spinal cord, a grade 4 astrocytoma was seen in cross section to have destroyed the complete cord. The entire long dimension of the tumor is not known; since only a portion of the spinal cord in this case was available to us we cannot positively exclude the presence of syringomyelia, although there was no indication of this condition in the material studied.

Case 18

A man 46 years old, 7 months before he died in 1941, and 2 weeks after an attack of mumps and orchitis, began to experience bilateral frontal headaches. These headaches at first developed once a week, but subsequently became progressive until they were constant. They were accompanied by nausea and vomiting. The patient said that at night his arms and legs occasionally jerked.

During the previous 25 years the patient had experienced several attacks of severe pain in the lower part of the back; the last attack had developed at about the same time the headaches commenced. Since that time the lateral aspect of the left leg had remained partially anesthetic.

Examination disclosed an area of diminished sensation over the lateral surface of the left leg, and bilateral papilledema which was graded 1 diopter. The protein content of the cerebrospinal fluid was 850 mg. per 100 cc., with only 11 cells per cubic millimeter.

Encephalography disclosed slight symmetric dilatation of the lateral and third ventricles. There was no evidence of obstruction or of a space-occupying lesion.

The patient was dismissed with the presumptive diagnosis of encephalitis.

A month after he had been seen at the Mayo Clinic he died at home.

Necropsy.   The brain was found to be swollen, but no other gross abnormalities were noted.

A fusiform swelling, 6 cm. long, was found in the spinal cord, extending from the middle part of the cervical segment to the level of the second thoracic segment. In a cross section a grayish tumor was detected in the center of the cord, extending into the surrounding tissue. In the levels of the cord above the tumor a cavity was present. The tumor had spread to the meninges and had extended down around the cord and up to the base of the brain.

Histologic Aspects.   The tumor appeared to be composed of rows of nuclei separated from each other by acellular spaces (Fig. 66), which contain many inter-

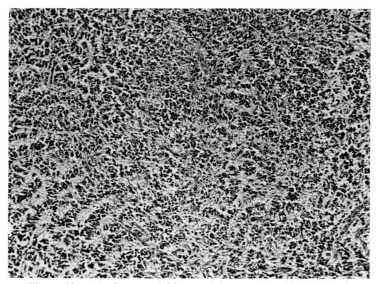

Figure 66. A "polar spongioblastoma" in case 18 in Chapter IV, showing tumor cells grouped in rows which are separated by acellular bands (hematoxylin and eosin; × 125).

woven, fibril-like structures, which did not stain blue with Mallory's phosphotungstic acid hematoxylin stain, and did not accept Holzer or Mallory-Heidenhain stains. Vessels could be discerned in these spaces; sometimes vacuolar spaces were present. The nuclei appearing in rows did not, for the most part, present any specific arrangement, but sometimes they exhibited a palisade-like structure. The cytoplasm was ill-defined and scanty. The nuclei were moderately pleomorphic (Fig. 67) and slightly irregular in staining intensity, some being clearly hyperchromatic. Mitotic figures were present but not abundant. In most areas the blood vessels, although increased in number, were thin-walled, but in some areas they showed slight endothelial swelling and proliferation.

At the level of the sixth cervical vertebra the tumor completely infiltrated the cord transversely. Above and below this site the tumor appeared to be located chiefly in one of the anterior horns; at various places it extended to the surface of the cord. The infiltrating quality of the tumor was apparent, and pre-existing

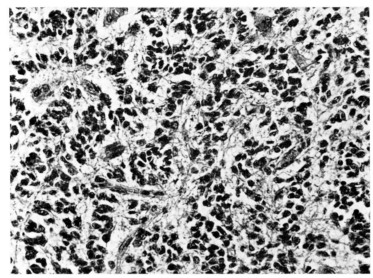

Figure 67. "Polar spongioblastoma," same case as in Figure 66. Slight nuclear pleomorphism and irregularity are evident; the cytoplasm is ill-defined and scanty (hematoxylin and eosin; × 300).

structures, such as ganglion cells and even the patent central canal, were found in the tumor mass.

The histologic structure of the tumor was not always the same. In several peripheral areas the lesion had the characteristics of a grade 2 astrocytoma. In these areas staining with Holzer stain demonstrated an increased number of glial fibrils.

The tumor extended along a cavity and formed part of the wall of the cavity. The remaining circumference of the cavity was composed of glial tissue similar to that of the wall of a syringomyelic cavity.

Parts of the tumor had a striking resemblance to the polar spongioblastomas described by Russell and her associate (1947,[245] 1955[244]), and while parts of this tumor differed from the other astrocytomas, we feel justified in classifying the lesion as a polar spongioblastoma in the sense conveyed by Russell and her associate. Since, however, part of the tumor had all the characteristics of an astrocytoma, we believe that some portions of the lesion would be classified with astrocytic tumors.

Conclusion. The history given by this 46-year-old man was unusual indeed, and appears to be atypical in respect to a tumor of the spinal cord. Discovery of the lesion at necropsy was a surprise. The unusual histologic aspects of the tumor also make the case outstanding.

EPENDYMOMAS

Case 19

A woman had been first seen at the Mayo Clinic in 1949, 10 years before her death at the age of 72 . For 8 months she had noticed a sensation of burning and tingling, with some pain, in the upper extremity, shoulder, and neck on the left;

numbness of the fingers and forearms and soreness of the shoulder on the right. Tingling awakened her from sleep.

At examination the index and middle fingers of the left hand were seen to be swollen, and the metacarpophalangeal joints were tender and warm. The palms of both hands were reddened, and a tremor was present which was most marked in the left hand.

The patient was thought to have osteoarthritis and was treated for that disease.

Six years later the patient returned. At that time she had a metastatic carcinoma of the breast. She was seen at regular intervals during the next 4 years, and only once during that period did she complain of temporary pain in the lower part of the thoracic region of the spinal column. This pain apparently cleared spontaneously.

Necropsy.   Carcinomatosis, with emaciation, was the cause of death.

The spinal cord contained two lesions: one 0.7 by 0.8 cm., in the midcervical region; and one 0.4 by 0.2 cm., in the filum terminale.

Histologic Aspects.   The cervical tumor was located in the area of the dorsal columns. It had partially infiltrated and partially pushed the dorsal horns laterad. There was an apparent loss of ganglion cells in both posterior horns, and the central canal area had been absorbed into the tumor. No remnants of the central canal could be recognized.

The tumor was a grade 1 ependymoma, moderately cellular, with a minimal degree of pleomorphism and no mitotic figures. The only remarkable feature of note was that the center of the ependymoma was completely hyalinized. This type of hyalinization is seen more frequently in ependymomas of the brain, and seems to be more rare in ependymomas of the spinal cord, although some of the latter sometimes have broad hyalinized septa. In most areas the tumor seemed to be fairly sharply demarcated from surrounding tissues, but it had no capsule. The line of demarcation was irregular, indented in some places and bulging in others, and in one place the tumor obviously was infiltrating the substance of the spinal cord.

Anteriad to the tumor (Fig. 61) were three small structures which appeared to be composed of Schwann cells and which most probably represented small neurilemmomas. Similar structures, for the most part, however, of smaller size, are not infrequently encountered in routine sections of the spinal cord, especially in the thoracic and lower cervical areas.

The tumor in the filum terminale also was a grade 1 cellular ependymoma. It was slightly more cellular than the lesion in the cervical region, but pleomorphism and hyperchromatism were not increased and mitotic figures were not seen. In one side of this was a small, slitlike cavity lined by cuboidal ependymal cells which represented an epithelial pattern in a cellular ependymoma.

Conclusion.   At the age of 62 years this woman was seen at the Mayo Clinic with symptoms in the upper extremities which were thought to be caused by osteoarthritis. At necropsy two independent ependymomas, one in the cervical portion of the spinal cord and one in the filum terminale, were found. It is possible that the former lesion, a slow-growing cellular ependymoma, was related to the patient's symptoms manifested 10 years before her death. In addition, there were three small intramedullary neurilemmomas.

Case 20

A 46-year-old man, 11 months before he was operated upon in 1921, complained of pain in the shoulders and feet, soon followed by attacks of vaguely localized pain which seemed to originate low in the abdomen and to terminate near the back of the neck. Two or three months later stiffness in the legs appeared, and 5 months after the onset of pain the legs suddenly gave way. After a remission, the weakness slowly but steadily progressed again. Six months after the onset of difficulty the patient noticed numbness in the legs and a tendency to stagger while he was walking. He was constipated.

Examination disclosed weakness in both legs, more pronounced in the left than in the right; the knee and abdominal reflexes were absent, the Achilles reflexes were slightly exaggerated, and Babinski's sign was elicited bilaterally. Complete anesthesia and nearly total analgesia were found to obtain from the third rib downward. Roentgenologic examination disclosed nothing of significance. Lumbar puncture produced straw-colored cerebrospinal fluid; the reaction of the Nonne-Apelt procedure was positive; the fluid contained 18 cells per cubic millimeter.

Exploratory laminectomy was done. It extended from the first to the third thoracic vertebrae. The dura was seen to be under considerable tension. After the cord had been split for a distance of about 8 cm., a purplish-red, partially encapsulated, granular tumor was exposed. A specimen was taken for biopsy, and the dura was left open.

Total paralysis of the legs and slight weakness of the left arm remained after the operation. Dermatitis developed, and urinary difficulty arose which necessitated frequent catheterization. Infection of the urinary tract, with orchitis and epididymitis, supervened, and the patient died 2½ months after the operation.

Necropsy.   Cystitis, ureteropyelonephritis, and terminal bronchopneumonia were noted.

At the level of the spinal cord between the second and third thoracic vertebrae was a protruding, irregular, soft, reddish tumor mass, about 4 by 1 by 1.5 cm. When the spinal cord was sectioned below this level a cavity was found which extended down to the lumbar enlargement. Above the site of the tumor was another cavity which was split in two at the upper end. There was also an area of softening in the left lateral region of the cord. The cavities were lined by a smooth, grayish, gelatinous substance about 0.5 to 1 mm. in thickness.

Histologic Aspects.   The tumor was identified as a moderately cellular grade 1 ependymoma. Pleomorphism and mitosis were not found. In several places thin clefts were seen which were lined by cuboidal ependymal cells. The tumor had completely destroyed the spinal cord at this level; normal structures of the spinal cord could not be recognized.

The portion of spinal cord directly above the site of the tumor appeared to be completely infarcted except for an area in the dorsal columns. We found a thrombus in one of the main branches of the anterior spinal artery.

In the subdural space, attached to the spinal cord, we observed an extension of the tumor.

The cervical segment of the cord contained two fairly small syringomyelic cavities. One of these was located on one side of the cord, between the base of the posterior horn and the median dorsal septum. The second cavity was situated slightly more anteriad and extended toward the opposite side of the cord. Both cavities were lined by a fairly thick layer of dense glial tissue, deficient in cells but abundant in neuroglial fibrils. In this wall many Rosenthal fibers were present. The walls of the cavities appeared to be connected at about the midline of the cord. One of the cavities had a focal lining consisting of a row of 10 to 15 ependymal cells. In the infarcted area of the cord no evidence of these cavities was to be found. The central canal could not be detected, but at the anterior borderline of the most ventrally located cavity and the normal portion of the tissue of the spinal cord we saw an interrupted row of groups of ependymal cells with a tiny rosette.

In that part of the spinal cord below the site of the tumor a single, fairly large syringomyelic cavity was found in the center of the cord. This cavity extended up to the level of the tumor; it was lined by a type of glial tissue similar to that of the lining of the upper cavity. In the midline of the ventral wall a small group of ependymal cells was found lining the cavity. Anteriad to the cavity and coursing along with it to one side was, again, an interrupted row of groups of ependymal cells, located at the borderline of the glial tissue and the normal tissue of the spinal cord.

Conclusion.   The clinical picture of progressive pain and later the muscular weakness is well explained by the presence of a grade 1 cellular ependymoma in the upper part of the thoracic segment of the spinal cord. Extensive syringomyelia apparently had not produced symptoms. The sudden paralysis of the legs, followed by a remission, probably resulted from an indirect effect of the tumor. The recurrent, slowly progressing weakness very likely was caused by the infiltrating tumor itself.

Case 21

A farmer 52 years old had noted, approximately 10 years before he was operated upon in 1933, the onset of sexual impotence and some difficulty in starting the urinary stream. Two years later numbness of the right calf developed, which had been followed gradually by slowly progressing weakness of the right foot and leg. A year later similar symptoms appeared in the left leg. These conditions slowly progressed; 6 years after the onset, incontinence of the bowel and bladder was present. When this patient was seen at the Mayo Clinic he was unable to walk, and he complained of pain in the left hip and in the spinal column at the level of the fourth and fifth thoracic vertebrae. Occasionally this pain would extend up and down the spinal column.

Examination disclosed nearly complete spastic paralysis of the legs and abdominal muscles, more pronounced on the left than on the right; there was also disturbance of sensibility for all modalities below the level of the nipples. Reflexes were hyperactive and Babinski's sign was elicited bilaterally.

Roentgenologic examination of the spinal column revealed scoliosis in the thoracic area.

There was no manometric response of the cerebrospinal fluid to jugular compression. The protein content of the cerebrospinal fluid was 400 mg. per 100 cc., and there were 14 cells per cubic millimeter.

Exploratory laminectomy was done; it extended from the first to the fourth thoracic vertebrae. There was no pulsation of the dura. Through an incision in the posterior fissure a reddish, jelly-like tumor 6 by 2 by 2 cm. was removed. At this level the spinal cord was simply a thin layer of tissue that had surrounded the tumor.

On the eighth postoperative day chills and fever developed. Pus began to discharge from the wound; culture of a specimen produced staphylococci. Culture of a specimen of blood produced the same organism. The patient died on the twenty-fourth postoperative day.

Necropsy.   Evidence of staphylococcic sepsis, with abscesses in the lungs, heart, kidneys, and prostate gland, was found. Acute cystitis and pyelonephritis also were noted. The liver contained several cavernous angiomas.

The infection at the site of the laminectomy did not extend intradurally, and there was no evidence of meningitis.

The spinal cord at the level of the surgical intervention appeared to be markedly destroyed, but there was no evidence of a remaining portion of the neoplasm. Syringomyelia extended from the first cervical to the fourth lumbar segments (Fig. 68); in some places it was multilocular, with septa between the cavities, and in other places only a single cavity was to be seen. The cavities were smooth walled. At the ninth thoracic level another small neoplasm was found.

A thin-walled cyst was found attached to the right fifth anterior thoracic nerve root. The cyst was 1 by 0.7 cm., and was located entirely within the dura.

Histologic Aspects. The surgically removed tumor was a grade 1 cellular type of ependymoma. In some areas oligodendroglioma-like cells were present, and they were continuous with the ependymoma.

In a section of tissue taken at necropsy from the operative area, the cord appeared to be collapsed, and the central area was filled with blood, gitter cells, and cellular debris. Only a small rim of tissue of the spinal cord remained, and it exhibited degeneration of the fiber tracts. An occasional nerve cell could be detected along the borderline of the cavity. A few small groups of ependymoma cells appeared to be remaining.

The syringomyelic cavity extended as far as the level of the first cervical vertebra, and in the upper extension it consisted of a very small oval cavity located in the base of the dorsal column. The cavity was distinctly separated from the area of the central canal, which was composed of a fairly large group of ependymal cells without a canal. The wall at this level was not as dense in glial fibrils as at the lower extension, and a number gemistocytic astrocytes were present.

At the level of the third cervical vertebra were three distinct cavities, located on one side of the spinal cord between the compressed and displaced dorsal horn and the bulging median septum. In a more distal location (the seventh cervical vertebral level) only one larger cavity remained, extending to both sides of the spinal cord. At all levels the situation of the cavities was posterior. The cavities were separated from the area of the central canal, which remained obliterated, although an occasional minute rosette was present.

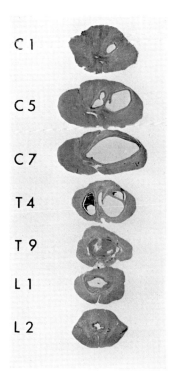

C 1

C 5

C 7

T 4

T 9

L 1

L 2

Figure 68. Case 21 in Chapter IV, showing syringomyelia with intramedullary subependymal glioma at the level of the ninth thoracic vertebra. A grade 1 cellular type ependymoma was removed from the spinal cord in the segment between the first and fourth thoracic vertebrae (hematoxylin and eosin; × 1).

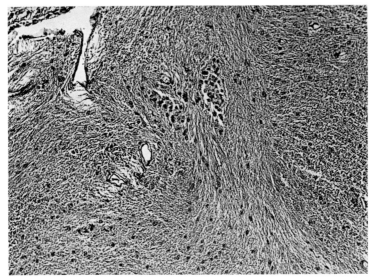

Figure 69. Subependymal glioma, same case as in Figure 68, showing fibrillar tumor with astrocytic type of nuclei and embedded groups of ependymal cells (hematoxylin and eosin; × 160).

Directly below the ependymoma, at the level of the fourth thoracic vertebra, were situated three cavities on either side of the spinal cord and separated from the central canal. These cavities, although they differed in number, shape, and location, persisted until the lower lumbar level. The walls of the cavities were composed of dense glial tissue in which Rosenthal fibers could be seen.

At the level of the ninth thoracic vertebra a structure which filled the central area of the spinal cord was found. This structure exhibited the characteristic features of a grade 1 astrocytoma, with numerous glial fibrils (Fig. 69) at the outer border of the tumor; however, groups of ependymal cells occasionally could be seen arranged around a minute canal. When Mallory's phosphotungstic acid hematoxylin and Holzer's stains were used, the glial fibrils stained specifically for astroglia. Within the tumor an irregular-shaped cavity was seen, partially clear but partially filled with a mass consisting of hyaline structures, blood vessels, and macrophages, a number of which were filled with brown iron pigment and some erythrocytes.

The tumor was almost completely separated from the surrounding tissues by a thin cleft in which many brown-pigmented macrophages and fresh erythrocytes were seen. The surrounding tissue consisted partially of moderately dense glial tissue similar to that of the lining of a syringomyelic cavity. Occasional Rosenthal fibers were evident. This tumor is a subependymal type of glioma (see Chapter II, "Intramedullary Gliomas of the Spinal Cord and Filum Terminale," p. 29.

At the same level of the cord, anteriad to the tumor, two small cavities were present. The walls of these cavities contained areas suggestive of a similar type of astrocytoma, and it appeared very likely that they represented an extension of the tumor.

Conclusion. It is difficult to determine which one of the pathologic anatomic findings was responsible for the various clinical symptoms in this case. The fully developed disease process appeared to have been dominated by the grade 1 ependymoma situated at the upper part of the thoracic segment of the cord, and the presence of this tumor excluded the possibility of recognition of lesions in the lower segment of the cord which may have been responsible for symptoms in the earlier phase of the disease.

Case 22

A farmer 46 years old reported the gradual development, over 9 to 10 years, of numbness and tingling in the feet and legs. Seven years later he experienced pain in the region of the second and third lumbar vertebrae which would awaken him at night, and which was so severe that he had to get up to obtain relief. A year later sensation in the legs was lost, and this was followed by weakness, particularly in the right leg.

At the Mayo Clinic this patient said everything seemed dead below a point midway between the umbilicus and the os pubis; the legs were spastic and weak. Coughing sometimes would produce momentary weakness in the knees to the extent that on one or two occasions he fell down.

Neurologic examination disclosed weakness in both legs; on the right paralysis was nearly complete. Reflexes in both legs were exaggerated; the abdominal reflex could not be elicited on the right; Babinski's sign was elicited bilaterally. Almost complete analgesia and thermal anesthesia were noted in many segments of both legs and over the lower part of the abdomen. Anesthesia extended over the soles of both feet. The gait was markedly ataxic.

The manometric response to jugular compression was slow. No other data were recorded.

Roentgenologic examination of the spinal column disclosed spina bifida occulta at the level between the fourth and fifth lumbar vertebrae.

Laminectomy was carried out (in 1926); it extended from the seventh to the eleventh thoracic vertebrae. The spinal cord was fusiform; enlargement was maximal opposite the ninth thoracic vertebrae. The cord felt cystic. After incision into the cord some brown fluid escaped and the cord collapsed. An intramedullary tumor was found and was partially removed.

On the eleventh postoperative day the patient suddenly died.

Necropsy. The cause of death was pulmonary embolism, originating in the left iliac vein.

The spinal cord was swollen, and the swelling was maximal in the region of the ninth thoracic segment.

Study of serial sections disclosed extensive degeneration in the posterior columns, in the spinothalamic tract, and also in much of the white matter on the right side.

At the level of the seventh thoracic vertebra cavitation was seen in the right side of the cord. Tumor tissue was first encountered at the level of the eighth thoracic vertebra; at the level of the ninth thoracic vertebra this tissue extended into both sides of the cord in the form of a circular mass of brownish-red, firm tissue which expanded the cord so that the cord appeared to be a thin layer, 1 mm. in thickness, surrounding the tumor.

At the level of the tenth and eleventh thoracic vertebrae the size of the tumor diminished, but some degree of cavitation was noted in this region.

Histologic Aspects. The cavity at the level of the seventh thoracic vertebra represented syringomyelia. The wall of the cavity was moderately dense neuroglial tissue. We did not find certain evidence of Rosenthal fibers. The cavity was located between the base of the dorsal horn and the median septum, and was dorsad to the central canal, which was composed of a group of ependymal cells.

The tumor at the level of the eighth to eleventh thoracic vertebrae was easily recognized as a grade 1 cellular ependymoma with a fairly extensive area in which the pattern was epithelial. In the center of the tumor an irregular-shaped hyaline mass was found which contained only a small number of nuclei. Around this mass a number of brown-pigmented cells were seen. The tumor was largest at the level of the tenth thoracic vertebra, and on one side it reached the sub-arachnoid space. The line of demarcation between the tumor and the surrounding part of the spinal cord was in some places clear-cut, but in several other places distinct invasion of the substance of the cord could be detected. At the level of the tumor we were unable to identify syringomyelia, but continuous with the tumor was a cavity lined in most places by several layers of ependymal cells. There was no evidence of a central canal at this level.

Directly below the tumor syringomyelia extended over about two segments of the central part of the cord; it was distinctly separated from the area of the central canal.

Conclusion.   In this case the slowly progressive symptoms of sensory and motor disturbance over a period of 10 years are well explained by the grade 1 ependymoma at the level marked by the eighth to the tenth thoracic vertebrae. Above as well as below the tumor a syringomyelic cavity was found.

Case 23

A man who was 26 years old in 1915 complained of persistent tenderness in the midlumbar region. He said the difficulty had been present for 5 years. During the 2 years preceding consultation soreness had developed in the lumbar region, and aching in both lower extremities became constant. He also experienced attacks of sharp, shooting pain in the posterior aspects of the thighs. These pains were worse at night. He also reported stiffness of the legs, retention of urine, and constipation.

At examination slight weakness of the legs and a saddle type of anesthesia for all modalities were noted. Reflexes in the legs were diminished, and Babinski's sign could not be elicited.

Lumbar puncture was done, but the result was a dry tap.

Roentgenologic examination of the sacrum disclosed that the laminae and spines of the first and second sacral vertebrae were absent. Erosion of the bones also was depicted.

Laminectomy was done; it extended from the eleventh thoracic to the fifth lumbar vertebrae. A tumor was found which extended even lower than this level. After a specimen had been taken for biopsy, the wound was closed temporarily because it was judged that a second operation would be performed.

On the second postoperative day high fever, convulsions, and signs of meningitis developed. On the fourth postoperative day the wound was re-opened. A considerable amount of pus was removed. The patient died the next day.

Necropsy.   Acute purulent meningitis was considered to be the cause of death.

The diameter of the spinal cord was seen to increase gradually from the level of the tenth thoracic vertebra downward. The spinal canal was widened; the diameter was 5 cm. at the level of the fourth lumbar vertebra. A tumor 14 by 5 by 2 cm. extended from the eleventh thoracic to the third sacral vertebrae; it was very soft and friable, and appeared to originate from the filum terminale.

Histologic Aspects.   The tumor was a grade 1 papillary ependymoma with a low degree of mucinous degeneration of the stroma, but many acini-like spaces were seen which were lined by cuboidal ependymal cells and filled with mucinous material.

The spinal cord was normal at all levels. The tumor expanded in the sub-arachnoid space and surrounded the nerve roots of the cauda equina and the lower portion of the cord but did not infiltrate these structures.

Conclusion. The clinical symptoms and findings are well explained by a grade 1 papillary ependymoma which originated in the filum terminale and completely filled the lower end of the dural sac, but which did not infiltrate pre-existing structures.

Case 24

A woman 23 years old said that left sacro-iliac pain had begun to be noticed 5 years prior to operation, done in 1933. This pain had become continuous, and was aggravated by her coughing and sneezing. It was worse at night, and she was unable to sleep in an extended position. Three and a half years later she began to suffer from cramps in the buttocks and thighs; the pain became more intense and extended around the lower part of the abdomen and down the backs of the thighs. There was also loss of sensation in the buttocks, backs of the thighs, and lower part of the abdomen. A year prior to the operation numbness developed in the calves and the soles of the feet, and weakness in the legs became apparent; she also suffered from retention of urine and loss of control of the anal sphincter.

Examination disclosed marked weakness and slight atrophy of the legs. Reflexes were completely absent. The gait was ataxic and spastic. There was also complete anesthesia for all modalities from the umbilicus down.

Roentgenologic examination of the spinal column showed obliteration of the shadows of the pedicles of the first to the third lumbar vertebrae and erosion of the spinal canal.

Exploratory laminectomy was done; it extended from the eleventh thoracic to the second lumbar vertebrae.* The lower end of the spinal cord was seen to be enlarged; below the conus a tumor was found which had originated from the filum terminale. A large portion of the tumor was removed from among the fibers of the cauda equina, and decompression was done.

On the fifth postoperative day a high fever developed, and the wound broke down and drained pus. Cyanosis supervened, and specimens of the cerebrospinal fluid were cloudy. Despite supportive measures the patient died on the tenth postoperative day.

Necropsy. The presence of spinal meningitis and bilateral bronchopneumonia was confirmed.

For the most part, the nerve filaments of the cauda equina were involved in a large tumor mass which extended from the level of the first sacral vertebra upward to surround the spinal cord to the level of the eighth thoracic vertebra.

Coronal sections of the cord revealed that the tumor did not involve the spinal cord itself, but surrounded it as a cuff. Marked cavitation was noted extending from the sixth thoracic to the fourth lumbar segment. Study of a longitudinal section through the lower end of the cord showed that the tumor originated from the middle portion of the filum terminale (Fig. 70) and that it was continuous with the tumor which encircled the cord. The tumor mass was grayish white, with multiple areas of hemorrhage.

Histologic Aspects. Microscopically, the tumor was a grade 1 papillary ependymoma with an occasional rosette formation. The cavitation represented syringomyelia, with a moderately dense gliotic wall of neuroglial fibrils. We found a fair number of swollen astrocytes, especially in the upper part of the tumor, and a moderate number of Rosenthal fibers which were more prominent in the lower

* Necropsy (see appendix) showed the lesion to occupy the region from the third to the fifth lumbar vertebrae.

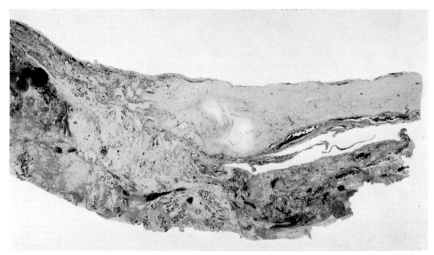

Figure 70. Grade 1 papillary ependymoma in case 24 in Chapter IV. The lesion originated in the filum terminale.

levels of the lesion. No ependymal cells lined the syrinx. The cavity did not extend into the sacral portion of the spinal cord, and it was not connected with the tumor; it involved both sides of the cord and was located between both dorsal horns and posterior to a group of ependymal cells.

At the level of the fourth thoracic segment was an area of recent softening which possibly was a progression of the syringomyelia, but this could not be determined.

Conclusion. The gradual development and the extent of the symptoms are in agreement with the finding of a grade 1 papillary ependymoma originating in the filum terminale. Syringomyelia extended from the sixth thoracic to the fourth lumbar segment, but had produced no obvious symptoms. The wall of the upper portion of the cavity appeared to be of more recent origin than the wall of the lower portions.

Case 25

A man 51 years old had been seen at the Mayo Clinic on many occasions for a variety of conditions unrelated to disease of the spinal cord. He died suddenly at home.

Necropsy. The cause of death was rupture of a dissecting aneurysm of the aorta.

Grossly, the appearance of the spinal cord was not remarkable.

Histologic Aspects. In the sections of the lumbar cord a small, grade 1 ependymoma was identified. It consisted of slightly pleomorphic ependymal cells located in moderately dense groups, sometimes with well-developed canal formation. Between the ependymal cells the subependymal glial tissue was increased. The tumor proper was sharply demarcated from the surrounding portion of the cord. A deep cleft appeared in the dorsal midline, in the area in which the dorsal septum normally is found.

Conclusion. A grade 1 ependymoma was found incidentally in the lumbar part of the spinal cord.

Case 26

A woman 62 years old was seen at the Mayo Clinic with a variety of diseases unrelated to disease of the spinal cord.

She died of the effects of chronic infectious arthritis.

Necropsy. Two whitish nodules, each 0.6 cm. in diameter, were found incidentally. They were attached to the filum terminale (Fig. 17).

Histologic Aspects. Both nodules were grade 1 cellular ependymomas. One of the nodules was composed chiefly of more spindle-shaped cells; the second one was constituted chiefly of polygonal cells with a slight degree of pleomorphism but no mitosis. In both a perivascular arrangement was seen. There was no separation between the nodules in the substance of the filum terminale; in fact, they appeared to be continuous.

Conclusion. A grade 1 cellular ependymoma attached to the filum terminale was found incidentally at necropsy.

Case 27

A man 62 years old was admitted to the hospital because of coronary arterial disease. He died shortly afterward of myocardial infarction.

Necropsy. Extensive myocardial infarction caused by coronary arteriosclerosis was disclosed.

At gross examination the spinal cord seemed to be normal.

Histologic Aspects. At the level of the fourth cervical segment of the cord an intramedullary, grade 2, cellular ependymoma was found. It was 0.3 by 0.2 cm. This tumor was located in the area of the central canal (Fig. 71). It extended to the anterior fissure and for a short distance into both of the anterior horns. Some degree of calcification was present in the tumor.

Invasion of the surrounding tissue by this neoplasm was clearly to be seen in several places, but in other areas the line of demarcation between tumor and other tissues was fairly sharp.

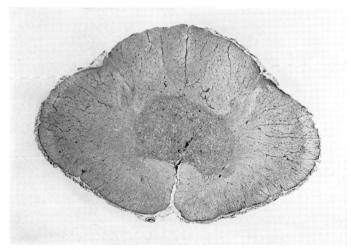

Figure 71. Section of the spinal cord in case 27 in Chapter IV. A grade 2 cellular ependymoma was found incidentally at necropsy (hematoxylin and eosin; × 7).

Conclusion.   A grade 2 cellular ependymoma was situated in the middle part of the cervical segment of the spinal cord.

Case 28

A man 40 years old was seen at the Mayo Clinic and treated for nephrolithiasis and muco-epidermoid carcinoma of the renal pelvis with metastasis. About 13 months before he died pain developed in the subscapular and paravertebral area and extended into the shoulders, but occasionally around the ribs or in the testicles. The pain was worse at night and often awakened him. The only neurologic finding at this time of examination was exaggeration of the reflexes in all four extremities. Four to 5 months before he died lumbar backache developed with extension to the posterior aspects of the legs.

Necropsy.   A muco-epidermoid carcinoma of the left kidney was found; there were many metastatic processes throughout the body. A retroperitoneal tumor mass was seen eroding through the lumbar vertebrae into the spinal canal, but it did not penetrate the dura. No gross abnormality was seen in the spinal cord.

Histologic Aspects.   Study of a section of the cord at the level of the fourth cervical vertebra disclosed a grade 2 cellular type of ependymoma, 0.5 by 0.3 cm. Moderate pleomorphism was seen, but mitosis had not taken place. The tumor was located approximately in the center of the spinal cord and reached the anterior fissure; for the most part it was sharply demarcated by a thin layer of relatively acellular gliotic tissue.

Conclusion.   The grade 2 cellular ependymoma discovered in the cervical portion of the spinal cord could explain the first period of pain, and the intraspinal but extradural metastatic process could be responsible for the last period of backache.

Case 29

In 1935 a man 44 years old experienced pain in the fourth and fifth fingers of the left hand. This pain gradually extended to the arm, and was associated with some degree of stiffness and weakness. Six months later the left leg was similarly involved, and some months later the right leg and right arm became affected in the same manner. In 1937 the gait of the patient became difficult and staggering, and he experienced aching and stiffness of the shoulders and back. He also noted muscular wasting and twitchings in the arms and legs.

Examination in 1937 revealed muscular weakness in both arms and upper legs, with atrophy of the arms. Reflexes in the arms were diminished; they were moderately exaggerated in the legs. Abdominal reflexes were absent. Sensory disturbance of varying intensity was most pronounced in both arms, the chest, and the upper part of the abdomen; it was exhibited to a lesser degree in both legs. The gait was ataxic, and Romberg's sign was elicited.

Roentgenologic examination of the spinal column revealed slight erosion of the right pedicles of the fourth and fifth cervical vertebrae.

Lumbar puncture disclosed complete block of the circulation of the cerebro-spinal fluid. The fluid was yellowish and contained 4000 mg. of protein per 100 cc.

Hemilaminectomy was carried out; it extended from the fifth to the seventh cervical vertebrae.* The spinal cord was greatly enlarged and felt cystic. It was incised, and an intramedullary tumor 2 by 3 cm. was gradually shelled out of its bed (subtotal removal). The dura was left open.

* Surgical exposure. Necropsy (see appendix) showed the lesion to occupy the region
    from the third to the seventh cervical vertebrae.

The postoperative period was satisfactory, but at the time of the patient's dismissal there was only slight improvement in the neurologic status.

When this patient was seen again in 1939, he reported only occasional pain in the back of the neck. Anesthesia extended to approximately the same level as previously, but it appeared to be less intense. He could walk with some difficulty without a cane, but he said that he sensed increasing weakness in the left foot and hand, an impression which was confirmed at the examination.

Roentgen-ray therapy was administered over the area of the cervical portion of the spinal cord.

At re-examination 3 months later no improvement was noted.

The patient returned 7 months later, in 1940, reporting a definite increase in symptoms. At that time paralysis of the left extremities was almost complete, and weakness of the right extremities was marked, with anesthesia extending from the nipples into the legs and on the medial sides of the arms.

Laminectomy was done again; it extended from the third cervical to the second thoracic vertebrae. A huge tumor was seen to occupy most of the spinal canal; it extended backward and laterad through the site of the previous laminectomy on the left. The entire tumor was shelled out. On the third postoperative day the patient became dyspneic and cyanotic and showed signs of pneumonia. His condition rapidly deteriorated, and he died on the fourth day after operation.

Necropsy. The cause of death was bilateral bronchopneumonia, with early formation of abscesses.

Gross examination of the spinal cord revealed the surgical defect extending from the third to the seventh cervical vertebrae. Study of transverse sections of the cervical portion of the cord, above the site of the tumor, demonstrated degeneration of the anterior columns. In addition, syringomyelia was seen to involve the cord from the level of the first cervical vertebra to the site of the surgical defect, and from the lower end of this defect to the first lumbar segment. The widest portion of the syrinx was 7 mm.

Two roots of the cauda equina were involved by tumor nodules measuring up to 2 mm.

Histologic Aspects. Sections of the tumor removed at both the first and the second operations were judged to be fairly cellular grade 2 ependymomas. No mitotic figures were seen. The specimen of the tumor removed at the second operation contained a few spaces lined by ependymal cells.

A section of the cord at the level of the tumor showed that only a small rim of cord tissue remained. Swelling of the fiber tracts was seen, and the nerve cells were degenerating. It did not appear that any of the tumor had remained after the operation.

In sections of the cervical portions of the cord above the site of the tumor a syringomyelic cavity was present, located posteriad to a well-marked central-canal area. The wall of this cavity was lined by moderately cellular glial tissue, and contained a fair number of gemistocytic astrocytes. The structure of this wall suggested that it was of recent origin.

Directly below the site of the tumor two cavities were found, but these apparently were joined to another at a slightly lower level. The walls of these cavities appeared to be denser, slightly less cellular, and without gemistocytic astrocytes. A few Rosenthal fibers were recognized. At most levels a group of ependymal cells were recognized located anteriad to the syrinx. Both above and below the site of the tumor fairly extensive degenerating areas were seen which contained numerous gemistocytic astrocytes. The nodules on the cauda equina were typical neurilemmomas.

Conclusion. A man 44 years old had a grade 2 cellular ependymoma in the cervical portion of the spinal cord which recurred after 2½ years, and syringomyelia which extended upward and downward in the spinal cord. In addition, there were two neurilemmomas in the cauda equina.

Case 30

In 1958 a woman 37 years old experienced a constant, burning discomfort over the right posterior iliac crest which spread gradually over the entire right leg and into the right flank, across the back and abdomen, and involved the left axilla and breast. About a year after the onset of this difficulty bilateral weakness developed in the lower extremities. On two occasions she had noted blurring of vision which cleared spontaneously.

When seen at the Mayo Clinic, this patient was affected by minimal weakness predominant in the left leg with marked hyperreflexia, more pronounced in the lower than in the upper extremities. Abdominal reflexes were absent, but Babinski's sign was elicited bilaterally. There was no disturbance of sensation.

Spinal puncture disclosed that the circulation of the cerebrospinal fluid was not blocked. The fluid contained 100 mg. of protein per 100 cc.

A myelogram made with Pantopaque showed swelling of the spinal cord at the level of the first thoracic vertebra, with well-developed obstruction.

Thoracic laminectomy was carried out between the first and second thoracic vertebrae. The spinal cord was purplish to the left of the midline. It felt cystic, but repeated punctures produced no fluid. The cord was incised, and a tumor was removed piecemeal.

On the fourth postoperative day the patient had difficulty with swallowing. She became unresponsive fairly rapidly, and although there were movements in the extremities, all the reflexes were diminished. Some hours later the patient died.

Necropsy.   The brain exhibited a moderate edema. The spinal cord contained a surgical defect at the level between the first and second thoracic vertebrae. Cross sections of the cord showed a remaining portion of tumor at the level of the seventh cervical vertebra and syringomyelia which extended two segments above and below the site of the tumor (Fig. 72). In addition, the spinal cord was fairly extensively degenerated above the site of the tumor.

Histologic Aspects.   The tumor was a grade 2 cellular ependymoma.

At the level between the seventh cervical and the first thoracic vertebrae several tumor nodules appeared to remain, and at the level of the second thoracic vertebra the spinal cord was infiltrated by tumor tissue so that several separate tumor nodules had developed at some distance from the original tumor.

Above the site of the tumor syringomyelia was present which, at the highest level, consisted of three small separate cavities which apparently united to form one cavity at a slightly lower level. Directly above the site of the tumor the cavity became much smaller again. Below the site of the tumor syringomyelia extended as far as the fourth thoracic segment, where it ended in an area of gliosis. The wall of the syrinx was composed of fairly dense glial tissue, with only a moderate number of nuclei. In the wall several Rosenthal fibers were recognized.

Syringomyelia affected the same side of the cord as that on which the tumor was located, and did not have any relationship to the area of the central canal, which was easily recognizable, except at the level of the tumor. At the lower end of the second thoracic segment of the cord an area was found in which ependymoma cells were found enclosed in tissue which partially resembled, in structure, the wall of the syrinx, although a cavity could not be seen at this level.

The remaining substance of the cord exhibited focal infarction and fairly extensive degeneration, with many gemistocytic astrocytes.

Conclusion.   A grade 2 cellular ependymoma, with syringomyelia, extended upward and downward for two segments in a 38-year-old woman who had had increasing sensory disturbance and paraplegia for 2 years.

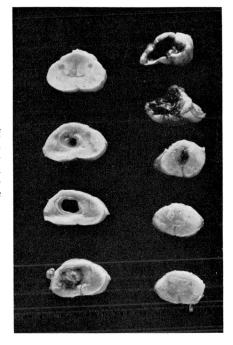

Figure 72. Transverse sections of the spinal cord in case 30 in Chapter IV. A grade 2 cellular ependymoma was situated at the level between the first and second thoracic vertebrae, and syringomyelia extended above and below the site of the tumor.

Case 31

A man 33 years old in 1951 began to notice difficulty with erection. Four months later progressive, dull backache began and extended into the right leg. The aching was aggravated by his coughing or sneezing. Seven months later weakness, stiffness, atrophy, and fasciculations developed in the right leg. Voiding also became increasingly more difficult.

When the patient was examined at the Mayo Clinic, marked weakness of the right leg was noted. Similar weakness, but to a lesser degree, affected the left leg. Reflexes in the right leg were almost entirely absent, and Babinski's sign could not be elicited. Abdominal reflexes were hyperactive. Marked atrophy of the right leg was evident. Areas of slightly disturbed sensation were found on the right leg, and saddle anesthesia was marked.

A roentgenogram of the spinal column disclosed rotary scoliosis in the mid-lumbar area, and widening of the neural canal with excavation of the posterior aspects of the vertebrae throughout the lumbar region. After lumbar puncture in the first lumbar interspace the manometric reaction of the cerebrospinal fluid to jugular compression was normal; the content of protein was 600 mg. per 100 cc., with 8 cells per cubic millimeter.

The Pantopaque myelogram showed a suggestive block of the radiopaque oil at the level of the first lumbar vertebra.

Laminectomy was done; it extended from the twelfth thoracic to the fifth lumbar vertebrae. This exposed a large, solid ependymoma arising from the filum terminale extending up to the level of the eleventh thoracic segment and filling the entire lumbar part of the spinal canal, ending at the level of the first sacral segment. The tumor had invaded some of the roots of the cauda equina and extended into the junction of the conus medullaris with the filum terminale. The impression of the surgeon was that he had removed all the tumor.

Two days after the operation the patient was seized by generalized convulsions which recurred on several of the ensuing days. The condition of the patient suggested that a subdural hematoma was present. This proved to be the case. At operation a fairly large subdural hematoma was removed.

Transurethral resection of the vesical neck and prostate gland was performed a month after the operation on the spinal cord.

At the time of dismissal the patient had mild rightsided hemiparesis and moderate sphincter dysfunction.

The patient returned 10 months later complaining of alternate numbness and tingling in the right foot and ankle, and some degree of weakness in the right leg. Examination disclosed anesthesia and moderate weakness in the right foot and lower leg. The patient received a course of roentgen-ray treatment.

He returned again 10 months later, reporting additional weakness which had affected both legs. Anesthesia of the right leg was extending.

The protein content of the cerebrospinal fluid was 500 mg. per 100 cc.

A myelogram made with Pantopaque was suggestive of block of the circulation of the cerebrospinal fluid at the level of the first lumbar vertebra.

The site of the laminectomy was re-opened. A tumor was not found, but extensive adhesive arachnoiditis was seen.

Sixteen days after this operation the patient was attacked by grand mal convulsions, and symptoms developed suggestive of a left cerebral lesion. A specimen of tissue was taken from the cerebrum through the trephine openings, and was reported as representing "degenerating brain."

A ventriculogram revealed dilatation of the ventricles. The presence of an obstructing lesion below the quadrigeminal plate could not be excluded. Left ventriculocisternotomy was done, but no obstruction could be visualized.

During the immediate postoperative course, the patient did fairly well, but a few days afterward several convulsions again supervened. The postoperative course was erratic, and after a convulsion the patient died, 48 days after the last spinal operation and 22 months after the first.

Necropsy.   Extensive bronchitis and bronchopneumonia were found.

The brain was edematous (weight, 2020 gm.), and a large, fairly recent infarct was noted in the left inferior medial occipital region. Another area of softening was seen in the right temporal lobe, involving the cortex. In the fourth ventricle granular ependymitis was detected.

In the area of the cauda equina a large, cigar-shaped tumor mass, grayish white and firm in consistency, was found extending from just below the conus for a distance of about 5 cm. The widest diameter was 2 cm. The spinal cord itself was enlarged and firm, up to the lower cervical region.

Histologic Aspects.   The tumor was a grade 2 ependymoma preponderantly of the papillary type, but it also contained areas in which the cellular type of ependymoma could be discerned. In a few places an epithelial-like arrangement was present.

The spinal cord was markedly edematous, but otherwise was not abnormal.

Conclusion.   A recurrent grade 2, predominantly papillary ependymoma was found in the lumbar area of the spinal cord. The tumor originated from the filum terminale.

OLIGODENDROGLIOMAS

Case 32

A woman 45 years old in 1943, and 15 months before death, experienced periods of pain and stiffness in the right side of the neck which were exaggerated by her coughing, sneezing, or movements of the neck. A year later the pain became constant and extended to the shoulder level and into the right arm. One month prior to operation numbness developed in both hands of the patient, gradually extending to the elbows. Sensory perception was decreased. Fourteen days before operation weakness began to be noticed in the right arm and leg; it increased gradually. Urinary retention and constipation had developed.

At the Mayo Clinic complete flaccid paralysis of the right arm and leg was found, as well as grade −2 to −3 weakness of the left arm. Reflexes were diminished in the arms, but were approximately normal in the legs. Anesthesia of grade −2 to −3 was noted in the right shoulder and upper arm, in the left leg, part of the left side of the abdomen, and the right leg below the knee.

A roentgenogram of the spinal cord revealed wide separation of the right pedicles of the third and fourth cervical vertebrae.

At spinal puncture complete block of the circulation of the cerebrospinal fluid was demonstrated. The fluid was xanthochromic, and the protein content was 2400 mg. per 100 cc., with 2 lymphocytes per cubic millimeter.

Right hemilaminectomy was done; it extended from the second to the fifth cervical vertebrae. An extraspinal and extradural tumor was found and removed. The dura was not opened.

On the tenth postoperative day thrombophlebitis developed, and on the twentieth postoperative day the patient became suddenly unresponsive, with very shallow respirations. Fluid was found in the right pleural space and was partially removed.

The patient died 24 hours later, of progressive medullary failure.

Necropsy. Bilateral bronchopneumonia with nonfatal pulmonary embolism was recorded. The brain apparently was normal. Anteriad to the spinal cord (Fig. 45), extending from the foramen magnum downward to about the level of the fifth cervical vertebra, a mottled, scarlet-red tumor was found, 2½ to 3 inches long. It lay parallel to the cord and was compressing it. The tumor was growing out of the cord.

Histologic Aspects. The tumor appeared to be an oligodendroblastoma with considerable pleomorphism but relatively few mitotic figures. As can be seen in Figure 46, the tumor originated from one anterior half of the cord at the level of the third cervical vertebra, and expanded intradurally. In most areas the tumor appeared to be fairly well demarcated, although there was no lining membrane, and in some places invasion of the substance of the cord was obvious.

The remaining portion of spinal cord appeared to be normal.

Conclusion. An oligodendroblastoma originating at the level of the third cervical vertebra had expanded extensively in the intradural and extradural spaces.

Case 33

A woman 29 years old in 1925, 20 months before she was operated upon, and at a time when she was 2 months pregnant, experienced pain of increasing severity in the back at about the lower sacral level. Five months later this pain extended along the course of the sciatic nerves and was especially troublesome at night, forcing her to arise from bed. The pain was aggravated by her coughing or sneezing, or by jarring movements. Temporary remission of the pain lasted 6 months, but 4 months before she was operated upon the pain increased again, and was accompanied by numbness in the right foot which later extended to the leg. Weakness developed in the legs, and difficulty with walking persisted for about 8 months. In the last few weeks prior to her examination at the Mayo Clinic difficulty was noted in her passing urine, and it was associated with constipation.

At the time the patient was examined at the Mayo Clinic it was noted that she was pregnant again. Moderate weakness (grade −2) and some degree of atrophy (grade +1) of the right leg were detected. Reflexes were absent in both legs except for a grade +1 knee jerk on the right. Hypesthesia of grades −1 to −2 was present in the right hip, upper part of the thigh, and foot. The patient reported a sensation such as would be caused by a band constricting the lower part of the thorax on the right. She also had saddle anesthesia.

At spinal puncture, complete block of the circulation of the cerebrospinal fluid was demonstrated. The fluid was yellow, and contained 6 lymphocytes per cubic millimeter.

Roentgenologic examination of the spinal column disclosed nothing abnormal. A myelogram depicted the column of Lipiodol as split from the fifth to the tenth thoracic vertebrae.

Laminectomy was carried out; it extended from the fourth to the eighth thoracic vertebrae. When the cord was split dorsally a cyst was found. It was opened. It contained yellow-brown fluid. A specimen was taken for biopsy, and the dura was closed.

The postoperative course was uneventful. At the time of dismissal the patient was walking well and reported very little difficulty from the type of pains previously experienced.

After the patient had been home for a month, the pain gradually began to return.

In a letter from the patient's home physician it was said that the patient had died 5 months after the operation.

She had given birth to a baby 3 weeks prior to her death, and at that time she apparently had been paralyzed from the waist down, with marked trophic disturbances of the skin.

Two weeks before her death her vision began to fail. She had papilledema of both eyes, as well as some degree of deafness.

Necropsy.   It was reported that no abnormalities were found in the brain or meninges. The spinal cord was sent to us for examination.

Cross sections of the cord revealed a tumor which extended from about the sixth thoracic to the second lumbar segments, entirely filling the inside of the cord and leaving only a small, narrow lamina of nervous tissue. At the level of the first lumbar nerve root the tumor encroached upon the meninges posteriorly. Above this level a crescent-shaped tumor mass involved the arachnoid over the posterior aspect of the cord.

Histologic Aspects.   The tumor was an oligodendroglioma with foci of oligodendroblastomas. In many areas the tumor obviously was infiltrating the surrounding tissues, but the zone of transition was rather narrow. The entire cord, up to the cervical area, was completely surrounded by tumor tissue in the arachnoid.

In the dorsal part of the cord, above the site of the tumor, up to the fourth thoracic level, a small, slitlike syringomyelic process was found, with a thin but fairly dense gliotic wall. The lower levels of the cavity had been replaced by tumor. Below this level the tumor filled the center of the cord; there was no syrinx. Below the site of the tumor a syringomyelic cavity again occupied the dorsal column area.

Conclusion.   An oligodendroglioma with foci of oligodendroblastomas was found extending from the sixth thoracic to the second lumbar segment, with syringomyelia above and below the site of the tumor.

VON RECKLINGHAUSEN'S DISEASE

Case 34

A man 20 years old was first seen at the Mayo Clinic in 1920, complaining of a protruding left eye, and difficulty in walking. For 6 years use of his hands had been impaired. At the age of 16 years he had experienced a severe attack of nausea, vomiting, and bilateral frontal headache associated with temporary blindness. The attack lasted 3 to 4 days, and since that time had been repeated each summer. At the age of 17 years he had noted wasting of the muscles of the left hand and forearm, inability to extend the little and ring fingers, and weakness of the adductor muscle of the thumb of that hand.

Two months prior to his visit to the Mayo Clinic he had noticed progressive difficulty in walking after dark, and numbness of the feet and legs. Just before the time of examination control of the sphincters of the bowel and bladder had been lost.

At examination multiple subcutaneous firm nodules were noted in the antecubital fossa of the right arm, on the left ulnar nerve at the elbow, near the head of the left calf muscle, and in the external peroneal nerve on the left side. A café-au-lait patch, 5 by 10 cm., was noted below the left nipple. Left-sided exophthalmos was found to be caused by a retrobulbar mass. Vision was diminished, and a papilledema of 2 diopters was detected in that eye.

Neurologic studies demonstrated diminished hearing on the left, with marked weakness and atrophy of the muscles of the left arm and forearm in the area supplied by the ulnar nerve. Weakness and atrophy also affected the interior tibial and peroneal muscles and the extensor muscle of the toes of the right foot. In addition, spastic weakness of all muscles and a diminished sensation for all modalities below the tenth thoracic segment were noted. Reflexes in the left leg were exaggerated, and Babinski's sign was elicited. The gait was ataxic, and Romberg's sign was produced.

At several operations neurofibromas were removed from the orbit of the left eye, right arm, and left leg. Laminectomy, extending from the sixth to the ninth thoracic vertebrae, exposed a meningioma, which was removed.

The patient improved remarkably. The gait became better, and the ataxia abated. He regained control of the sphincters of the bladder and rectum, and the sensory loss in the lower extremities was markedly reduced in extent.

Fourteen months after dismissal the patient was reported to be entirely well. The left eye had been enucleated for cosmetic reasons.

The patient returned in 1923 with persistent hoarseness of 3 months' duration and twitchings in the right hand associated with tingling in the two medial fingers of 15 months' duration. He had had several generalized convulsions.

Neurologic examination disclosed marked weakness of the left hand; moderate weakness of the right hand and leg was noted. All reflexes were diminished. The gait was ataxic. The left vocal cord was fixed. Funduscopic examination of the right eye demonstrated papilledema of 2 diopters. The right ulnar nerve was moderately enlarged, and contained a nodule in the cubital groove.

No therapy was instituted. The patient returned 2 years later with increasing numbness from the umbilicus downward and inability to walk without crutches as a consequence of increased weakness of the legs. Difficulty in moving the bowels and in starting the flow of urine had increased.

Re-examination revealed, in addition to the foregoing, moderate weakness of the right lower abdominal muscle group and the right leg and, to a somewhat lesser extent, the left leg. All reflexes were diminished, on the right more than on the left. Marked incoordination in the legs and moderate anesthesia below the umbilicus were found. Elevation of the choked disk at this time was 3 diopters.

Laminectomy was carried out from the sixth to the eleventh thoracic vertebrae. The cord was seen to be markedly swollen, and contained an intramedullary tumor, a specimen of which was taken for biopsy.

Two months later intracranial exploration was performed. Part of a meningioma in the left temporal region was removed.

The patient went home, but his general health deteriorated and he died 8 years after he was first seen at the Mayo Clinic. His brain and spinal cord were sent to us for examination.

The gross examination of the dura and cord revealed many meningiomas of varying sizes. Histologically, the tumors were of the meningothelial and psammomatous types. A large (5 by 3 cm.) acoustic neurilemmoma was found on the right, and a small neurilemmoma was detected on the left.

In the spinal cord three distinct swellings were observed: in the midthoracic, upper, and lower lumbar areas. The other portions of the spinal cord appeared to be atrophic. Almost every nerve root exhibited one or more small swellings which on histologic examination appeared to be neurilemmomas.

Study of cross sections through the spinal cord showed three distinct intramedullary tumor masses in the areas corresponding to the gross swellings.

Above the site of the tumor in the midthoracic portion of the spinal cord, as well as between that location and the tumor in the upper part of the lumbar segment (and also below the level of this latter tumor), syringomyelia was seen to involve the center of the cord. The upper pole of the upper lumbar tumor had a rounded end which projected into the syringomyelic cavity. The upper and lower limits of the syringomyelic process extended in the form of gliosis in the center of the cord. The wall of the cavities had a gelatinous appearance.

In the medulla oblongata a fairly large ependymoma (diameter 7.5 mm.) was found which did not extend into the cervical portion of the cord. In most areas the tissue of this tumor exhibited a gradual transition into the tissue of the medulla oblongata, but in a few places it was fairly sharply demarcated and appeared to be bordered by condensed glial fibrils.

Histologic Aspects.   All three tumors of the spinal cord were identified as cellular types of ependymomas, grade 1. The one in the upper part of the lumbar segment of the cord was the largest; it had about completely destroyed the pre-existent tissue of the spinal cord.

Except for the tumor in the upper part of the lumbar segment of the cord, the tumors had a fairly indistinct line of demarcation with the surrounding tissues, and this consisted mostly of zones in which the tumor was infiltrating. The pre-existing structures were more or less recognizable. At the levels of the tumors we were unable to detect the ependymal cells of the area of the central canal. They were present in areas of the spinal cord located between levels of the tumors, and were clearly separated from the syringomyelia. The central canal itself was obliterated.

The wall of the syringomyelic process was composed of a zone of condensed neuroglial fibrils with only a few cells present. A few Rosenthal fibers were seen. The syringomyelia was located just dorsal to the center of the cord, involving the anterior part of the dorsal columns and extending on each side for a minor distance into the base of the posterior horns.

Conclusion.   Apart from numerous neurilemmomas and meningiomas, we found three intramedullary ependymomas (and one in the medulla oblongata) with syringomyelia which extended from the second thoracic to the lower lumbar levels.

Case 35

A man 28 years old was first seen at the Mayo Clinic in 1937. He gave a history of increasing difficulty with hearing of 8 years' duration, weakness and atrophy of the interossei muscles of the right hand of a year's duration, difficulty in walking at night, and headache that gradually had become continuous and of increasing severity. Also noted was a "tendency to numbness."

At examination firm tumor nodules were detected in the region of the ulnar nerve of the right upper arm, at the level of the lower third portion of the fibula, in the region of the junction of the right first metacarpal-carpal bones, under the left internal malleolus, and at the inner canthus of the right eye. Neurologic examination demonstrated slight nystagmus, bilateral nerve deafness, atrophy of the interossei muscles of the right hand, diminished knee and Achilles reflexes, slight ataxia, and a subjective decrease in sensation of pain on the right half of the body.

Bilateral papilledema of 2 diopters was recorded.

Roentgenograms of the skull revealed tumors of the eighth cranial nerves, bilaterally. Roentgenograms of the thoracic segment of the spinal column showed compression of the body of the eighth thoracic vertebra, which was interpreted as post-traumatic.

Bilateral suboccipital craniotomy was performed; a neurilemmoma was removed from each eighth cranial nerve. On the left side there was also a neurilemmoma of the ninth cranial nerve; this lesion also was removed.

At the end of the first postoperative day the patient's temperature increased and the pulse slowed; he became cyanotic, the respiration ceased, and he died.

Necropsy. The cause of death was determined as edema of the brain and brain stem.

The brain and dura were found to be normal except for slight dilatation of the ventricles.

Many neurilemmomas were present: in the third, fifth, eighth, ninth, tenth, eleventh, and twelfth cranial nerves; in the thoracic and abdominal sympathetic nerves; in the intercostal and in many peripheral nerves; in the esophageal wall and in many dorsal roots and fibers of the cauda equina (Fig. 73).

The spinal cord appeared to be markedly enlarged at the levels of the fifth and sixth cervical segments, second to fourth thoracic segments, and at the sacral area.

Study of cross sections at these levels revealed intramedullary neoplasms. Extending for two or three segments above the tumor in the cervical segment was a syringomyelic process.

Histologic Aspects. The upper two tumors were grade 2 ependymomas. They were composed predominantly of elongated cells with moderately large, oval nuclei which presented a mild degree of pleomorphism but no mitosis. Except for the perivascular arrangement, there were no other characteristic arrangements.

In sections stained with hematoxylin and eosin many cells appeared to contain fibrils, but generally these fibrils did not accept the Mallory phosphotungstic acid stain or the Holzer stain.

The tumor in the sacral level was similar to the upper two tumors, except that in certain areas polygonal cells, easily recognized as classical ependymal cells, were present. Part of the tumor, stained with Mallory's phosphotungstic acid stain and with Holzer's stain, exhibited more fibrils staining as astroglia than did the two tumors located higher anatomically. It is our experience that the presence of fibrils which have the same staining characteristics as astroglia does not contradict the diagnosis of ependymoma. In all three tumors we discerned ample evidence of blepharoplasts. In many areas the tumor tissue was

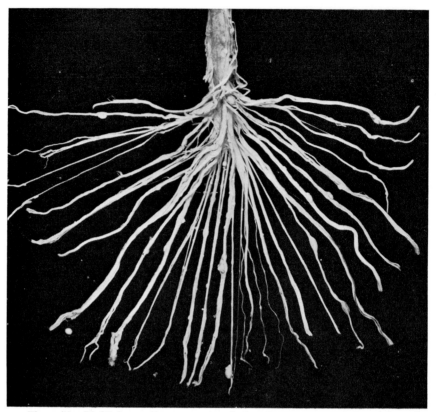

Figure 73. Multiple neurilemmomas attached to the nerve roots of the cauda equina in case 35 in Chapter IV.

fairly distinctly separated from the normal tissue, but in a few areas infiltration appeared to have taken place. The normal structures were distorted, and this was especially true of the gray matter, which seemed to be compressed to a small rim between the tumor and the remaining tissue of the cord. Ganglion cells were still easily recognizable at the junction of the tumor, but they appeared to be less numerous.

The wall of the syrinx above the site of the upper tumor was composed of varying concentric rings of glial fibrils. The cell content of the outer layers was higher than that of the inner ones. Rosenthal fibers were easily recognized, but they varied in frequency of occurrence in several locations. The syringomyelic process was located in the dorsal half of the cord, and had almost completely replaced the dorsal columns. Syringomyelia descended into the area of the tumor. The tumor was found anteriad to the cavity and extended laterally around, but outside, the wall of the syrinx, almost completing a ring around it. There was no area in which the tumor appeared to be lining the cavity. The wall of the syrinx was easily separable from the tumor; both appeared to be separate entities. At this level there was no central-canal area, although such an area was found at the higher level in which no tumor was present; it was located anteriad to the syringomyelic process.

Conclusion.   A man 28 years old had Von Recklinghausen's disease, three intramedullary tumors of the spinal cord, and syringomyelia.

Case 36

A girl 10 years old was first seen at the Mayo Clinic in 1922. She limped, and manifested weakness and atrophy of the right leg which was more pronounced in the distal part and which had developed within the preceding year. Reflexes on the right ranged from normal to grade +1; on the left the range was from grade −2 to −4. The cerebrospinal fluid was normal. No cause for the weakness and atrophy of the leg could be determined.

A brace was prescribed for the patient, but no change in the condition was apparent in the years following.

The patient returned at the age of 23 years after she had been involved in an automobile accident. She had sustained fracture, without displacement, of the second cervical vertebra and had been treated successfully with traction exerted on the neck. The paralytic condition of the right leg previously noted appeared to be essentially unchanged.

A few months after the accident small tumors were removed from the occipital region and from the scalp. These tumors had been regarded as neurilemmomas.

Four months after the accident orthopedic correction was performed for hallux valgus and hammer toes on the right foot.

The patient was seen again at the age of 27 years. At that time she had ataxia and difficulty in walking, especially in the dark. The Romberg maneuver revealed a tendency to fall to the left; marked lateral and slight vertical nystagmus was recorded. The patient had tinnitus on the right and hearing loss, more marked on the right than on the left. The muscles of the right shoulder were atrophied, and a mass was present in the right part of the upper portion of the thigh. This mass, at biopsy, proved to be a neurilemmoma.

Bilateral cerebellar craniotomy was performed. On each side intracapsular enucleation of a neurilemmoma at the cerebellopontine angle was done. After the operation loss of hearing was nearly complete, and right-sided paralysis of the facial nerve ensued for the relief of which the spinal accessory nerve was anastomosed with the facial nerve.

The condition of the right leg and the ataxia remained essentially unchanged. Romberg's sign continued to be elicited.

Nothing was heard from the patient until a few days before her death 4½ years later. Paralysis had gradually increased, and the vision diminished. She was unable to walk and had lost nearly all the use of her arms. She experienced difficulty in swallowing and breathing. The eyes protruded. Shortly after she was admitted to a hospital she lapsed into coma and died. She was 32 years old.

Necropsy. A horseshoe kidney was found with a few fibroleiomyomas in the capsule.

The intracranial and the intraspinal dura was found to be studded with numerous small, firm, round, encapsulated nodules varying from 0.2 to 3.5 cm. in diameter. They were attached to the inner surface of the dura and were indenting the surface of the brain and spinal cord. Some of the tumors were pedunculated; others appeared as small seeds implanted in the meninges.

At the base of the right side of the cerebrum a soft, yellowish necrotic tumor was found which had grown around and over the tuberculum sella and which filled half of the medial part of the middle fossa.

A large tumor mass was found to be herniating through the left side of the tentorium cerebelli, pushing the entire pons and medulla past the midline to the right. This mass appeared to be attached to the temporal bone; it was firm and well encapsulated.

Histologic Aspects. All these tumors were found to be varying types of meningiomas (meningothelious and psammomatous).

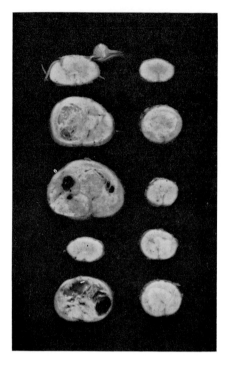

Figure 74. Case 36 in Chapter IV. Von Recklinghausen's disease. Four separate intramedullary tumors and a small neurilemmoma attached to the second cervical posterior nerve root (same case as that in Figure 1).

Neurilemmomas were found in both third cranial nerves, both seventh and eighth cranial nerves, and in the sciatic nerve and the brachial plexus.

Cross-sectioning of the brain disclosed a tumor in the substance of the right frontal lobe. This lesion also appeared to be a meningioma.

Three marked swellings were seen in the spinal cord (Fig. 1), but study of serial sections disclosed four intramedullary tumors (Fig. 74) (in the cervical, high and low thoracic, and lumbar segments of the cord). A fifth tumor was present in the filum terminale, and neurilemmomas also were attached to the nerve roots of the spinal cord. Syringomyelia was not detected.

Histologic Aspects. Examination of the spinal cord and filum terminale revealed that all the tumors were fairly classical examples of grade 1 cellular ependymomas. The diameter of the cervical tumor was 1.7 cm.; that of the tumor in the upper thoracic segment was 1.2 cm.; that of the tumor in the lower thoracic segment was 0.9 cm.; that of the tumor in the lumbar segment was 0.7; and that of the tumor in the filum terminale was 0.6 cm. in the longest dimension. A few cysts were found in the two tumors of the upper part of the cord; some of the cysts were completely surrounded by tumor tissue, others were partially lined by tumor tissue, and some were partially lined by fairly normal spinal-cord tissue. The nontumorous wall did not resemble the structure of the wall of a syrinx, and we regard these cavities as the results of edema or of breakdown of tumor tissue or secretion by the tumor cells.

In all sections the tumors were centrally located in the substance of the spinal cord, and were covered by it nearly everywhere. The architecture of the spinal cord was completely distorted, and at levels at which tumors occurred no central-canal cells could be found. The gray matter was found chiefly at the borders of the tumors, and it was obvious that the number of ganglion cells was decreased.

The gray matter was not only pushed laterally, but often was infiltrated by the tumor cells. In several other areas the tumor was sharply demarcated, and occasionally gliosis appeared bordering the tumor.

Segments of the spinal cord between the tumors were normal.

One additional observation worth mentioning is that in several sections of the left frontal lobe areas were found which contained small groups of highly malignant astrocytes. Most of the groups were still very small, but they were multiple, and we consider them to be the early phase of a grade 3 or grade 4 astrocytoma. They were also encountered in the gyrus rectus, internal capsule, and parietal area.

In both this case and case 5 the tendency toward multifocal formation of tumors is similar.

Conclusion. This was an instance of Von Recklinghausen's disease in which with many meningiomas and neurilemmomas, four intramedullary ependymomas, an ependymoma of the filum terminale, and an early phase of a multifocal astrocytoma in the brain had developed.

Case 37

A boy 12 years old was seen for the first time at the Mayo Clinic in 1951. Clubfoot had been noticed when he began to walk. At the age of 6 years right facial palsy developed, which had abated since that time. Two months before his visit to the Mayo Clinic he manifested weakness in the right arm, and the right foot began to drag. Enuresis and urinary incontinence had been present for 4 weeks.

At the clinic right spastic hemiplegia of grades −3 to −4 was detected, and right peripheral facial palsy was observed. Reflexes on the right were slightly exaggerated.

Ventriculography disclosed moderate dilatation of the lateral ventricles and no filling of the third ventricle.

Results of examination of the cerebrospinal fluid were essentially negative.

Right suboccipital craniotomy and bilateral cervical laminectomy were performed. A multicentric meningioma was removed from the right cerebellopontine angle, the foramen magnum, and the upper two cervical segments of the spinal cord.

Postoperatively there was much improvement in the strength on the right side of the body, but the facial palsy persisted.

The patient returned 7 months later with tinnitus, increasing deafness in the right ear, and slight loss of sensation of pain and temperature at the lateral surfaces of both feet and the first two fingers of the right hand.

Two and a half years later he gradually became unable to control his right leg and could walk only with difficulty. Weakness of the right arm was evident, and atrophy of these extremities had occurred. A "lump" had developed above the right ear.

At examination the weakness and atrophy were confirmed. Marked ataxia was demonstrated, but sensory disturbances were not.

No therapy was instituted.

When this patient was seen again, 9 months later, increasing weakness of the left hand was seen, and there was a questionable area of minimally disturbed sensibility around the abdomen. Marked scoliosis of the thoracic sector of this spinal column had developed.

The sites of the suboccipital craniectomy and the cervical laminectomy had to be reopened for subtotal removal of a recurrent meningioma. At the time of the patient's dismissal weakness was still considerable, and a minor degree of impairment of sensibility of both right and left upper extremities remained. Reflexes in the right upper and lower extremities and the left lower extremity were slightly exaggerated, and in the left upper extremity they were slightly diminished.

Four months after the operation the patient was seen again. He complained of pains all over the body. There was not much change in his condition except that the reflexes in the right arm had become diminished to grade −2 to −4.

In his home city the patient had received a series of cobalt 60 treatments without benefit.

Seven months later complete urinary incontinence and severe spasm of the right leg developed.

Examination demonstrated marked increased paralysis in all four extremities and decreased sensation below the level of the fifth thoracic vertebra. The patient was unable to stand or walk. The left twelfth cranial nerve also was involved. A course of roentgen-ray therapy was administered to the suboccipital and high cervical regions.

We were informed by letter that during the last months of his life and 3 months after his last visit to the Mayo Clinic the patient had been completely bedridden and had lost the sight of the right eye.

The patient died at home. The last days of the life of this 18-year-old boy were marked by many convulsions.

Necropsy.   This examination was performed elsewhere. The pathologic report and material were sent to us by Dr. Arnold K. Myrabo, of Sioux Falls, South Dakota. We found numerous tumor masses attached to the dura of the brain and spinal cord. The right optic nerve was embedded in such a tumor. These tumors had indented the brain and spinal cord. Histologically they were identified as meningiomas, mostly of the psammomatous type. Neurilemmomas were attached to several nerve roots.

In the lumbar sections of the spinal cord a tumor was found which was located anteriad to a syringomyelic cavity. This cavity extended above and below the tumor.

Histologic Aspects.   The tumor appeared to be a grade 1 ependymoma that was partially infiltrating the outer wall of the syrinx, but had not entered the cavity itself. There was no central canal at this level. The syringomyelic process consisted of one section of three different cavities.

The walls of all these cavities were similarly composed of a moderately dense, glial fibril network with only a small number of cells; Rosenthal fibers occasionally were present. They were separated from a distinct area of the central canal. In one of the dorsal areas was a huge neurilemmoma which fused completely with the tissue of the spinal cord. The arachnoid was absent between the tumor and the substance of the cord. It is possible that this lesion was an intramedullary neurilemmoma, but the evidence is uncertain.

Conclusion.   This was an instance of Von Recklinghausen's disease with, in addition to numerous meningiomas and neurilemmomas, an intramedullary cellular type of ependymoma and syringomyelia.

VASCULAR TUMORS

Case 38

A man 48 years old experienced, in November, 1931, 10 months before his death, attacks of severe pain at the upper portion of the neck, just under the occiput. The pain extended from that area to the frontal region. These attacks were preceded by episodes of dizziness, during which he would fall to the left. The episodes lasted only several minutes, and were brought on by change of position or jarring of the head.

The patient also was seized with hiccup, which at first had been only occasional, but which had become more or less constant in the 3 to 4 months preceding his visit.

At night he sometimes experienced cramps in the legs, followed by a sensation of numbness.

Examination disclosed slight nystagmus, grade −2 Achilles reflex bilaterally, and a grade +1 ataxic gait. Papilledema of 1 to 2 diopters was noted.

The protein content of the cerebrospinal fluid was 4000 mg. per 100 cc.

Surgical exploration was carried out through a cerebellar approach. A vascular tumor was found arising from the floor of the fourth ventricle and extending downward into the medulla oblongata. The tumor was nine-tenths cystic. As much as possible of the lesion was removed.

Some hours after the operation the patient experienced respiratory difficulty. The blood pressure gradually failed, and the patient died 12 hours after the operation.

Necropsy. Several carcinomas (hypernephromas) of both kidneys and multiple cysts in the pancreas were found.

The cerebrum was slightly edematous, and grade 1 dilatation of the ventricles was noted. The medulla oblongata was swollen, and the lower portion of the floor of the fourth ventricle exhibited the surgical lesion. In the right hemisphere of the cerebellum a smooth-walled, sharply circumscribed cyst was present; it was 3 cm. in diameter and contained a small tumor nodule about 10 by 7 mm. in diameter.

The upper part of the cervical portion of the spinal cord was involved by syringomyelia which extended downward for three segments and upward through the medulla oblongata to communicate with the floor of the fourth ventricle.

Histologic Aspects. Both tumors—the one in the cerebellum and the one surgically removed from the medulla oblongata—were hemangio-endotheliomas. At the lower end of the syringomyelic process, at the level of the third cervical vertebra, a third very small hemangio-endothelioma was found in the anterior wall of the syrinx.

The syrinx itself was composed of a fairly dense layer of glial tissue, containing only a few nuclei and occasional gemistocytic astrocytes. At several places small Rosenthal fibers could be recognized.

At the level of the upper cervical segment of the cord the axis of the cavity lay in the anteroposterior direction, but in the lower level the axis was laterally directed.

Conclusion. This was a fairly typical instance of Lindau's disease with multiple hemangio-endotheliomas in the cerebellum, medulla oblongata, and spinal cord, and with syringomyelia, syringobulbia, and a cyst in the cerebellum. In addition there were cysts in the pancreas and multiple carcinomas (hypernephromas) in both kidneys.

Case 39

In 1930 a man 20 years old experienced numbness in the tip of the right fourth finger; this difficulty gradually extended up the entire right arm. In 1936 he noticed weakness in the same extremity. At the same time pain developed in the back of the neck and upper part of the shoulder during coughing, sneezing, and straining at stool. In 1937 he was operated upon elsewhere, and an inoperable "glioma" of the cervical part of the spinal cord was found. Five months after the operation weakness began to be evident, associated with slight numbness of the left arm and muscular atrophy which seemed to originate in the shoulder. The right leg was slightly spastic. In the ensuing months the patient received a series of roentgen-ray treatments.

When this patient was seen at the Mayo Clinic in June, 1940, marked weakness of both arms and, to a lesser degree, of both legs, was noted. A sensory disturbance of varying degree (more pronounced on the right than on the left) was present from the neck down. Reflexes in the arm were diminished, but were exaggerated in the legs.

No therapy was given until the patient returned 4 months later. At that time the muscle weakness in the legs had progressed, and control of the bowels had been lost.

Spinal puncture demonstrated complete block of the circulation of the cerebrospinal fluid; the protein content of the fluid was 400 mg. per 100 cc., with only 1 lymphocyte per cubic millimeter.

The site of the laminectomy wound (third to the fifth cervical vertebrae) was re-opened. It was seen that most of that part of the spinal cord at the level of the site of laminectomy was involved by an infiltrating lesion. Especially noted was a markedly increased vascularity of the entire cord at this level. A specimen was taken for biopsy.

Postoperative complications were respiratory difficulties and paralysis of the arms and legs. The patient died 7 days after the operation.

Necropsy.   Extensive bronchopneumonia with formation of abscesses was seen. The kidneys and pancreas, like the brain and cerebellum, were normal. The medulla oblongata was involved by syringobulbia which extended to the upper part of that structure and which distally was continuous with syringomyelia in the cervical portion of the spinal cord. In the segment marked by the third to the sixth cervical vertebrae the spinal cord was completely replaced by a solid hemorrhagic tumor (Fig. 75). Distal to the tumor syringomyelia featured by numerous cavities extended down to the lower lumbar level. From the mid-dorsal region to the lower lumbar level of the spinal cord there apparently was only one cavity with only a thin shell of tissue of the cord.

Histologic Aspects.   The tumor was a hemangioblastoma which had almost completely destroyed the spinal cord and which contained a large, fresh hemorrhage. In the distal extension the tumor was encountered in the dorsal half of the spinal cord posteriad to several large cavities filled with blood. These cavities did not have distinctive walls. One cavity, however, contained only a few erythrocytes, and the wall of the cavity was composed of a small rim of gliotic tissue not unlike that of the syringomyelic process.

All the cavities above and below the site of the tumor were typical syringomyelic cavities with walls of dense glial tissue in which many Rosenthal fibers were found. At several levels multiple or separated cavities appeared to be present.

At all levels, except at sites at which the tumor was too extensive, we found a central-canal area with ependymal cells.

Conclusion.   In this case, in addition to the presence of a hemangioblastoma, that part of the spinal cord above and below the site of the tumor was extensively involved by syringomyelia.

Case 40

A woman 30 years old came to the Mayo Clinic in May, 1925. Five years earlier, after a fall, she had experienced a sensation of numbness from the neck down. This sensation had lasted for an hour. She said she had had some difficulties with weakness and dull pain in the back since that time. Ten months prior to her visit to the Mayo Clinic she had been afflicted with acute abdominal pain for which appendectomy had been performed. After that she could not walk as well as previously because of progressive weakness and paresis of the left leg and, to a lesser extent, of the right. The pain in the back had become constant and was located more on the left than on the right.

Physical examination revealed a low abdominal mass.

Neurologic examination demonstrated weakness of grade -2 with spasticity of the left leg, weakness of grade -1 in the left arm, and slight weakness in the right leg. Reflexes in the arms were normal, but in the legs they were all exaggerated, and Babinski's sign was elicited bilaterally. Sensation for all modalities was disturbed, most markedly in the upper part of the trunk, but also in both legs and the inner side of both arms. Slight nystagmus was detected. A roentgenogram of the spinal column disclosed nothing abnormal.

At spinal puncture complete block of the circulation of the cerebrospinal fluid was discovered. Reaction to the Nonne-Apelt procedure on the cerebrospinal fluid was positive. The fluid contained 6 lymphocytes per cubic millimeter.

Exploratory laminectomy was carried out; it extended from the second cervical to the second thoracic vertebrae. The spinal cord was three times normal size; it was soft and covered with numerous tortuous vessels. Only a decompression operation was done.

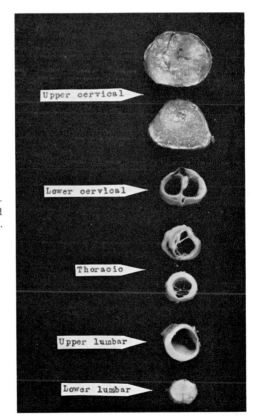

Figure 75. Spinal cord with intramedullary hemangioblastoma and syringomyelia, case 39 in Chapter IV.

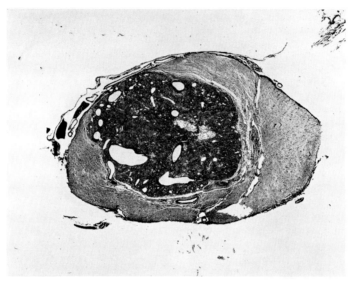

Figure 76. Spinal cord with intramedullary hemangioblastoma, case 40 in Chapter IV (hematoxylin and eosin; ×5½).

On the fourth postoperative day the patient's temperature increased suddenly and cyanosis developed. The patient died on the sixth postoperative day.

Necropsy.   Several hypernephromas were found in both kidneys, and multiple cysts were seen in both kidneys and in the pancreas and lungs. A metastatic hypernephroma was found in the omentum.

The cerebrum was entirely normal, but on the inferior surface of the right lobe of the cerebellum a nodule 7 mm. in diameter was found which extended into the cerebellum for 5 mm.

The spinal cord was swollen diffusely at three anatomic levels: from the third to the sixth cervical segments; from the eighth cervical to the second thoracic segments (Fig. 76); and at the eighth thoracic segment. At the first two levels the cord appeared to be soft and reddish. At the level of the eighth thoracic segment the cord fluctuated. On the posterior surface of the twelfth thoracic segment a small, elevated nodule 3 mm. in diameter was found. Study of cross sections of the cord disclosed multiloculated syringomyelia.

Histologic Aspects.   Four hemangioblastomas were detected: one in the cerebellum; one at the level of the second to fifth cervical segments; one at the level of the first and second thoricic segments; and one on the outside of the spinal cord at the level of the twelfth thoracic segment. The remaining portion of the cord was involved by syringomyelia as far upward as the medulla oblongata and downward to the lower lumbar level. The wall of the syrinx was not so dense in glial fibrils as is usually seen, and it also appeared to contain more cellular elements and nuclei. Rosenthal fibers were readily found.

The hemangioblastomas had sharp lines of demarcation next to the tissue of the spinal cord, and the lesions were not surrounded by gliosis. At the levels of the cord involved by tumors syringomyelic walls could be found, but at the poles the tumors appeared to be projecting into the cavity.

Conclusion.   In this case four hemangioblastomas were involved. Two were located in the substance of the spinal cord and were associated with syringomyelia; the third was situated on the outside of the cord; the fourth had developed in the cortex of the cerebellum and was not associated with a cyst. In addition, several hypernephromas with metastasis and cysts were found in the kidneys, pancreas, and lung. There were no hemangiomas in the retinas.

Case 41

A man 32 years old noticed in 1933, 5 years before his visit to the Mayo Clinic, a sharp pain in the neck when he made sudden movements. Shortly afterward numbness developed in the hands which was followed by pain in the upper part of the thorax when he coughed, sneezed, or strained. At examination at this time it was noted that the left eye was blind. Two years previously progressive incoordination of the hands had become apparent.

Examination disclosed minimal weakness and diminished sensibility in both arms, more pronounced in the right than in the left. All reflexes were slightly exaggerated; incoordination was marked, and the gait was ataxic. Papilledema of 6 diopters was found in the right eye, and an angioma was observed in the left eye. A roentgenogram of the spinal column disclosed nothing abnormal, but a roentgenogram of the skull revealed signs of increased intracranial pressure.

Bilateral suboccipital craniotomy was performed, with laminectomy of the upper part of the cervical sector of the spinal column. A large hemangioma, completely filling the fourth ventricle and posterior cistern, was discovered, and cysts were seen in the cerebellum and upper part of the cervical segment of the spinal cord. Subtotal removal of the tumor was done.

The patient died during the next night, after considerable respiratory difficulty.

Necropsy. Multiple cysts were found in the pancreas and kidneys, and several adenomas were encountered in both kidneys.

The brain was slightly edematous, and the ventricles were moderately dilated. The right retina exhibited two hemangio endotheliomas, and the left retina, one hemangio-endothelioma. A residual tumor mass also was found in the right cerebellar hemisphere.

The lower end of the medulla oblongata and the upper portion of the cervical segment of the spinal cord appeared to be hemorrhagic and infarcted.

The entire spinal cord appeared to be thickened. Study of cross sections disclosed a cavity which was continuous from the cervical to the low lumbar area. In the upper part of the lumbar segment of the cord, part of the cavity was filled by a vascular tumor.

Histologic Aspects. The cerebellar tumor and the tumor of the spinal cord were hemangioblastomas.

The cavity was typically syringomyelic. The wall was composed of dense glial tissue containing Rosenthal fibers. That portion of the spinal cord outside the syrinx at places appeared to be edematous. In the upper part of the lumbar segment of the cord the hemangioblastoma was attached to the dorsal wall of the cavity and projected into the lumen of the cavity. Rosenthal fibers were especially numerous at this level. At all levels a distinct central-canal area was found with a patent central canal.

At a level two segments below the site of the tumor, in the same location as the syrinx, a gliotic area was found. The center was loose and edematous, and was surrounded by a band of dense gliotic tissue in which a few Rosenthal fibers were seen.

Conclusion. In this case all the typical components of Lindau's disease were present with, in addition, syringomyelia and an intramedullary hemangioblastoma.

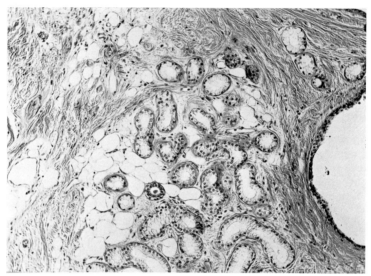

Figure 77.   Intramedullary teratoma in case 42 in Chapter IV. Glandular structures, fat tissue, connective tissue and part of a cyst lined by epithelial cells are seen (hematoxylin and eosin; × 100).

TERATOMAS

Case 42

A man 67 years old was seen at the Mayo Clinic on several occasions because of conditions unrelated to disease of the spinal cord. He died suddenly at home from the effects of a penetrating duodenal ulcer and gastrointestinal hemorrhage.

Necropsy.   In the sacral segment of the spinal cord a swelling was found; it was approximately 2.5 cm. in length. There was no connection between this swelling and the surrounding dura. Longitudinal sectioning showed the swelling to be cystic in some areas and soft, gelatinous, and yellow in others.

Histologic Aspects.   The tumor was a teratoma which contained tissue components of all three germinal layers (several types of epithelium were found which lined mucus-filled cysts, sweat glands [Fig. 77], connective tissue, fat tissue, and nerves). In most sections the tumor was separated from the tissue of the spinal cord by a rim of connective tissue. At the upper pole, however, was a small syringomyelic cavity in close connection with the tumor, not separated from it by connective tissue. The wall was composed of dense glial tissue with a fair number of Rosenthal fibers. There were no signs of malignancy.

Conclusion.   A teratoma was found incidentally at necropsy in the sacral part of the spinal cord. There also was a syringomyelia.

COMMENT

We had 33 cases available for more detailed anatomic and histologic study. Eight of the lesions were astrocytomas, one was a spongioblastoma,

13 were ependymomas, four were examples of Von Recklinghausen's disease complicated by intramedullary ependymomas, two were oligo-dendrogliomas, four were vascular tumors (of which three exhibited the other manifestations of Lindau's disease), and one was a teratoma.

We had several more cases in which a vascular malformation (angi-oma) was found. These examples are not included in this study, since they are not neoplasms, although we realize that they can cause symp-toms. Most, however, appeared to be silent, and represented incidental findings at necropsy.

In 19 of the 33 cases in which necropsy was done syringomyelia was associated. The incidence of this condition as associated with intra-medullary tumors of the spinal cord is given in Table 25. It appears

Table 25. *Incidence of Syringomyelia: 33 Cases of Intramedullary Tumor of the Spinal Cord in Which Necropsy Was Done*

Lesion	Cases	Syringomyelia Found
Astrocytoma	8	3
Spongioblastoma	1	1
Ependymoma	13	6
Von Recklinghausen's disease	4	3
Oligodendroglioma	2	1
Vascular tumors	4	4
Teratoma	1	1
Total	33	19

that the frequency of occurrence of syringomyelia and such lesions in the groups in question varies between 37.5 and 100 per cent, the average in our total series being 57.6 per cent. In 53 of the surgical cases the presence of a cavity in the spinal cord was noted at the time of opera-tion, and in 26 instances we found histologic evidence suggestive of the wall of a syringomyelic cavity. It is thus rather obvious that syringo-myelia constitutes an important problem in relation to tumors of the spinal cord, and this problem justifies more detailed study and descrip-tion.

Although there is no general agreement on the point, we define syringomyelia as "a cavitation in the spinal cord which appears pri-marily unrelated to the central canal and which has a wall composed of glial tissue which does not exhibit evidence that the cavitation is the result of hematomyelia or myelomalacia." At least, on theoretical grounds, syringomyelia should be distinguished from hydromyelia, which to us means dilatation of the central canal, the walls of which are at least partially lined by ependymal cells. A syringomyelic cavity can expand into and incorporate the cells of the central canal, thus becoming partially lined by ependymal cells and being then, at that site, indistinguishable from hydromyelia.

The development of syringomyelia is still a matter of considerable controversy. Existing theories can, according to Wilson[303] (1940), be considered either on a congenital or on an acquired basis. To the two groups of investigators, each of whom defends one of these theories, can be added a third whose opinion it is that syringomyelia is not one entity but simply the end-phase resulting from more than one pathologic process. According to Schlesinger[258] (1902) and Berkwitz[19] (1934), the oldest report of a cavitation in the spinal cord dates to 1564, and was given by Etienne ("Estienne," according to Tamaki and Lubin[281] [1938]). Later descriptions, also according to Schlesinger[258] (1902), came from Brunner (1688) and Morgagni (1740).

Ollivier (1824), cited by the same authors,[19, 258] introduced the term, "syringomyelia." It was his opinion that persistence of a patent central canal represented an abnormal feature. Stilling (1859) argued that patency of the central canal was normal, and that syringomyelia was the result of dilatation of this canal.

Hallopeau[114] (1870), cited by Tamaki and Lubin, suggested that the primary lesion in syringomyelia was sclerosis in the region of the central canal. Simon (1875) described the cavitation as resulting from softening of "gliomas" in the spinal cord.

Leyden[171] (1876) thought that syringomyelia was a developmental disorder subsequent to disturbance of the closing mechanism of the primitive spinal cord.

Langhans[164] (1881) suggested that syringomyelia resulted from congestion.

Schultze (1882,[259] 1885[260]) propounded the idea that syringomyelia resulted from a subsequent breakdown in an area, with abnormal development and growth of ependymal cells.

In 1902 Schlesinger[258] published the second edition of his monograph. That the nature and origin of syringomyelia were already controversial subjects at that time can be concluded from his being able to collect more than 1100 references from the literature. His own opinion was that syringomyelia is not one etiologic entity but one which can result from numerous causes. Some of the possible factors he referred to were: developmental anomaly, breakdown of congenital (?) central gliosis, trauma, neoplasm, vascular alterations and occlusion, increased intracranial pressure, and infection.

During the subsequent years all these factors have been supported by some and attacked by other investigators.

Bielschowsky and Unger[21] (1920), Henneberg and Koch[120] (1923), and Bremer[29] (1929) supported the theory of the congenital origin of syringomyelia, and Bielschowsky and Unger expressed the idea that acquired syringomyelia does not exist. Bremer brought to attention the constitutional, familial, and hereditary factors (status dysraphicus) which he thought might be involved.

Tamaki and Lubin[281] (1938) concluded from their study: ". . . that syringomyelia, *sui generis,* is a developmental anomaly, caused by imperfect formation of the central canal by primitive medullary epithelium. Resultant cell rests later undergo gliosis. Cavitation in the poorly nourished gliotic tissue is an end result of the process. Syringomyelia is therefore a heterotopic and benign process, which may be differentiated histologically from tumor formation by the lack of characteristic proliferative and invasive gliosis."

Tannenberg[282] (1924), Tauber and Langworthy[284] (1935), and Netsky[201] (1953) related the development of a syrinx to vascular anomalies and to vascular insufficiency which ultimately might result in an inadequate blood supply.

The role of infection in the development of syringomyelia was suggested by Hallopeau[114] (1870) and by Joffroy and Achard[134] (1887). Later this notion was expanded and supported by Jonesco-Sisesti[138] (1929) and by Levaditi, Lépine and Schoen[169] (1929).

In a monograph Staemmler[270] (1942) presented a critical review of the existing theories about the origin of syringomyelia and tested them against the observations in 24 cases of his own. His final conclusions about the histogenesis of syringomyelia embodied 12 points: the main idea is that fluid from the central canal escapes into the surrounding tissue of the spinal cord and causes a swelling of the glial tissue, liquefaction and dissolving of the nervous tissue, and proliferation of glial elements. The basic change for this process, in his opinion, is dysraphy.

The frequency of occurrence of the combination of syringomyelia and an intramedullary tumor of the spinal cord also is, in his opinion, greater than could be expected on a fortuitous basis. He wrote that he would accept such instances of syringomyelia as exceptional ("Sonderfällen"), and he thought he had found some acceptable grounds for his conclusions in the mechanism of development as detailed by Kirch[154] (1928).

In his study, Kirch divided syringomyelia into two groups. What he called "intrablastomatöse Syringomyelie" is not syringomyelia at all, but is simply a cyst within a tumor. What he describes as "extrablastomatöse Syringomyelie" would be accepted on the basis of present-day criteria for the identification of syringomyelia. He regarded a disturbance of circulation, with serous transudation, as the important factor in the development of the cavity. Edema, he thought, develops in the tumor as well as in the surrounding tissue. The beginning of the formation of edema is said to take place in dilatation of the lymph vessels; within these vessels transudates form which proceed to the perivascular lymph spaces. The edema is said to spread into the neighboring tissue of the spinal cord in a longitudinal manner ("Stiftförming"), as is believed to occur in hematomyelia. The theory is that this spread causes cleavage of the substance of the spinal cord and infiltration of the surrounding tissues. Next, it is held, the pressure of the edema fluid causes secondary proliferation of the neuroglia, which is characterized by the great number and the parallel arrangement of the fibrils. The presence of Rosenthal fibers also is noted. The development of the solid glial strands is explained by the suggestion that the edema does not cause cleavage within the tissue, but rather, that the edema remains diffuse but still able to cause reactive glial proliferation. The reactive gliosis of syringomyelia and the development of the cavities are regarded as processes analogous to the formation of cysts around tumors in the brain and cerebellum.

Kirch recognized that the foregoing interpretation of this mechanism can provide an explanation only for those instances in which a tumor is present, and he recognized the possibility of "congenital" syringomyelia.

Jonesco-Sisesti[138] (1929) considered, in addition to the possibility of myelitis as a cause of cavitation, the notion that intramedullary tumors may arise from embryonic cell rests, and that syringomyelia could result from degeneration. He evidently was not sure whether the gliosis is the result or the cause of the degeneration.

Russell[243] (1932) and Wolf and Wilens[305] (1934) considered the syrinx more as the result of anemia and hemorrhagic softening, although the former author wrote that "the evidence is not conclusive."

Mackay and Favill[189] (1935) regarded syringomyelia and intramedullary tumor of the spinal cord as diverging manifestations of the same proliferative process in which the tumor represents simply a more actively proliferative process in the same glial elements which are responsible for the syringomyelia.

Liber[172] (1937), in a study on the nature of Rosenthal fibers, originally wrote that he found these fibers to be present only in cases in which there was an accompanying intramedullary tumor. But shortly afterward, Liber and Lisa [173] (1937) observed Rosenthal fibers in the wall of a syringomyelic cavity in the absence of a neoplasm.

In 1956 Poser[217] published the findings of a study of 234 cases in which syringomyelia was found at necropsy to be associated with a neoplasm of the central nervous system. In this series there were 186 intramedullary tumors, and in 155 of these cases the relationship between the tumor and the syrinx was known. In only 11.3 per cent of these cases was there no relationship between these two conditions. The tumors were both primary and secondary and, according to the histologic data presented, they belonged to 15 groups. On the basis of his study the author concluded ". . . that syringomyelia and its associated central nervous system neoplasms can best be explained on the basis of congenital anomalies resulting from faulty closure of the dorsal raphe with glial or mesodermal inclusions at the site of the faulty closure or at other locations in the central nervous system. The neoplasm and the syrinx are then the result of faulty differentiation, possibly a process similar to the one that in its extreme form results in one of the phakomatoses."

In our study we were interested in ascertaining whether or not we could detect a histologic difference in the composition of syringomyelia in cases in which an intramedullary tumor of the spinal cord was or was not present. For this reason we compared the histologic findings in six cases of syringomyelia without a tumor with the 19 cases in which we found syringomyelia associated with an intramedullary tumor of the spinal cord.

Our impression is, however, that the differences which we noted were matters of gradation only.

Most of the syringomyelic cavities in both groups appeared to be located at or in the base of the posterior columns or in the dorsal horn. In all these cases the syringomyelia appeared to be independent of the area of the central canal, which usually was located anteriad to it.

In syringomyelia the wall of the cavity is composed mainly of glial tissue (Fig. 78) which is extremely abundant in neuroglial fibrils that stain specifically with Mallory's phosphotungstic acid and with Holzer's stain (Fig. 79). The density of the glial fibrils is variable, and it is not unusual to find that the area adjacent to the cavity appears to be more loose (edematous?) in structure than the outer areas (Fig. 80). Occasionally the gliotic wall seems to be composed of concentric rings of glial

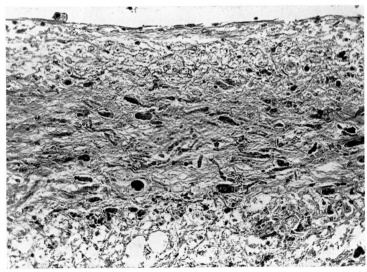

Figure 78. Wall of the cavity in syringomyelia, with moderate gliosis and several Rosenthal fibers (hematoxylin and eosin; × 225).

tissue with different densities of the fibrils. The arrangement of the glial fibrils does not appear to be specific, and the fibril may course in any direction, from one which is parallel to the wall to one which arranges the fibrils in a position at right angles to the wall. The thickness of the gliosis appears to be extremely variable; it was our impression that the wall generally was thicker in the cases in which there was a combination of syringomyelia with an intramedullary tumor.

In an occasional instance gliosis which exceeded the normal astroglial density of the gray commissure was not clearly recognizable, even with the aid of special stains. In some of these instances it was then noted that the lining of the cavity was formed by a row of ependymal cells which were independent of the central canal, or that the wall was composed of more "acute" astrocytic gliosis which contained a varying number of swollen and gemistocytic astrocytes. There remained, however, a few cases in which the wall appeared as normal tissue of the spinal cord, without any apparent reaction.

The nuclear content in the gliosis generally was low; it increased chiefly toward the outer layers of the wall. Mitosis was never observed, and there were no characteristics which would indicate neoplastic activity.

In a few cases of syringomyelia, both with and without a neoplasm, we noted the presence of a thin connective-tissue membrane on the inner wall of the syrinx; this, however, never extended around the whole circumference. Fragments of connective tissue either lying free or projecting into the syrinx, and containing one or a few blood vessels, were sometimes seen.

It is often noted in the literature that there is an increase in blood vessels in the vicinity of syringomyelia, and that these blood vessels often exhibit a hyaline thickening, calcification, or endothelial proliferation. Although we could observe this phenomenon in several cases, we do not feel that it can be accepted as reflecting a general tendency or that it bears any causative relationship to syringomyelia.

The presence, nature, and significance of the Rosenthal fibers is a much-debated problem. These structures were first observed and described by Rosenthal[239] in 1898 in a case of intramedullary tumor associated with syringomyelia. He described them as strongly glistening objects, shaped like small clubs or twisted sausages, with one end thick and the other tapering. The largest fibers appeared to be somewhat layered, as in amyloid bodies, but they gave no reaction to iodine. At times they seemed to be constituted of two parts: an outer hull which stained as glial fibers would stain, and a central part which stained with the hematoxylin lakes. It was Rosenthal's opinion that these structures represented degenerative glial fibers.

Bielschowsky and Unger[21] (1920) suggested the name, "Rosenthal fibers," and their opinion was that these structures are cytoplasmatic

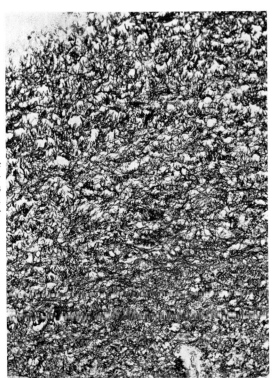

Figure 79. Wall of the cavity in syringomyelia, showing moderately dense gliosis with an occasional Rosenthal fiber (left lower corner) (Holzer stain; × 225).

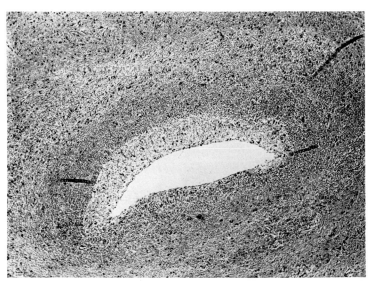

Figure 80. Syringomyelia, showing the varying density of the gliosis around the cavity (hematoxylin and eosin; × 75).

processes of glial cells which have retained their embryologic myelin-building function. In the following years these structures have been found in several conditions other than syringomyelia, such as in cerebellar astrocytomas [Landau[162] (1911) ; Bergstrand[18] (1937) ; Bucy-Gustafson[36] (1939)], in the subependymal gliosis around cysticercosis [Opalski[206] (1934)], in spongioblastomas [Zülch[314] (1940); Ringertz-Nordenstam[232] (1951); Henschen[121] (1955)].

Several studies have been made to detect the nature of Rosenthal fibers. Liber[172] (1937) suggested that they contain an iron-bearing hemosubstance. Grcevic and Yates[109] (1957) observed that the fibers exhibit a marked affinity for iron hematoxylin, acid fuchsin, and acid dyes, and that they are relatively easily impregnated with silver and gold. They found no evidence of the presence of carbohydrate, free lipid, amyloid, or iron, but the strong coupled tetrazonium reaction suggested a high content of protein.

Liber[172] (1937) and Grcevic and Yates[109] (1957) observed that the Rosenthal fibers appeared to be absent from the wall in cases in which syringomyelia was not accompanied by an intramedullary tumor. Liber and Lisa[173] (1937) reported, however, a case of syringomyelia, not accompanied by an intramedullary tumor, in which they found Rosenthal fibers.

We also observed Rosenthal fibers in their classical form of carrot-shaped, sometimes tortuous, bodies, which yielded a homogeneous, purple, eosinophilic reaction to hematoxylin and eosin. The form appeared to be variable, probably because of the way the fibers are sectioned. Sometimes they appeared as rounded structures which could be confused with amyloid bodies. In an occasional fiber we noted the presence of a nucleus, and other fibers were seen to taper to a small, elongated fibril of the thickness and character of neuroglial fibrils.

When several of our special stains were used, a number of the fibers did not appear to be homogeneous, but seemed to be layered or to have the appearance which an outer coating would impart (Mallory-Heidenhain stain) .

We used many special stains, but they did not yield any information additional to that already published by others. We believe that Rosenthal fibers have at least a relationship to astrocytes, and this belief is strengthened by the observation that the fibers also were found in a number of astrocytomas of a low grade of malignancy, but not in any other tumor.

Moreover, it is of interest to note that Rosenthal fibers are commonly found in the wall of the cavity in cases in which syringomyelia is associated with an intramedullary tumor of the spinal cord, whereas they are rare in cases of syringomyelia not accompanied by a neoplasm. In only one case of syringomyelia without a neoplasm did we find a suggestion of Rosenthal fibers. The frequency of occurrence of the fibers appeared

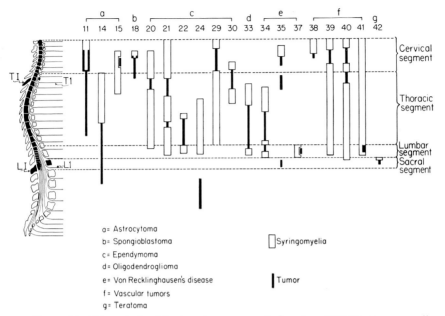

a= Astrocytoma
b= Spongioblastoma
c= Ependymoma
d= Oligodendroglioma
e= Von Recklinghausen's disease
f= Vascular tumors
g= Teratoma

☐ Syringomyelia

❚ Tumor

Figure 81. The relationship, based on anatomic location, between syringomyelia and intramedullary tumors of the spinal cord in 33 cases in which postmortem examination was done.

to be variable; in some cases they were abundant, and in others only a few could be found.

In all cases except one there appeared to be close association between the intramedullary tumor and syringomyelia (Fig. 81), and in several cases the tumor was either protruding into the cavity or forming part of the wall of the cavity.

The question whether an intramedullary tumor of the spinal cord has a causative influence on the genesis of syringomyelia remains open to doubt, but the frequency with which this combination occurs leads to suspicion in this respect. Conversely, the question might be asked whether syringomyelia is the forerunner of a tumor (whatever the mechanism may be). Nevertheless, it is remarkable that syringomyelia in the presence of an intramedullary tumor of the spinal cord remains silent, and is only rarely diagnosed clinically. What seems incontestable is the premise that there are several conditions which can lead to the formation of syringomyelia. Our impression, however, is that increasing thickness of the gliosis and the presence of Rosenthal fibers are more commonly observed in the association of syringomyelia with an intramedullary tumor than when syringomyelia without an intramedullary tumor is present.

V

Summary

This study is based upon 301 primary intramedullary tumors of the spinal cord and filum terminale which were observed at the Mayo Clinic during a period of 40 years. The lesions in 269 of these cases were classed as gliomas; 29 lesions were nongliomatous, and four were examples of Von Recklinghausen's disease complicated by one or more intramedullary tumors of the spinal cord.

It appears that about one of every 15 gliomas of the central nervous system was located in the spinal cord or filum terminale, and that primary tumors of the spinal cord and filum terminale constituted 22.8 per cent of all the primary spinal tumors.

In the medulla spinalis, considered in the strict sense, astrocytomas were found to be the tumors of most frequent occurrence, closely followed in this respect by ependymomas. Oligodendrogliomas constituted only a small group; in two cases a subependymal glioma was found, and in one case a polar spongioblastoma was found. It is concluded that on the basis of comparison of weights as between the brain and the spinal cord, astrocytomas and oligodendrogliomas occur in identical frequency in both structures, but that ependymomas have a tendency to develop in the spinal cord, and that they occur much more frequently than would be expected.

Slightly more than a third of all the tumors originated from the filum terminale, and 93 per cent of the tumors in this location were ependymomas.

In a review of the symptoms and signs it appears that no single symptom is diagnostic of an intramedullary tumor of the spinal cord. Pain appeared to be the most common sign; it was present in 68 per cent of our cases. It was especially interesting to note that pain almost invariably was present when the lesion was a tumor of the filum terminale. It

190

is also suggested that the asymmetry, anatomically speaking, of the extent and severity of the symptoms is an important guide to diagnosis. Among the more unusual signs of an intramedullary tumor of the spinal cord is bilateral papilledema, which was found in nine of our cases.

Among the laboratory examinations myelograms made with contrast media and determinations of the protein content of the cerebrospinal fluid appear to be extremely helpful aids in establishment of the diagnosis. The first procedure indicates, by evidence of blockage or distortion of the oil column, the presence and the level of a space-occupying lesion, and the second procedure often shows that the protein content of the fluid is markedly elevated without an increase of the cells.

Astrocytomas are divided into the four grades of malignancy according to the criteria indicated by one of us (Kernohan) and associates[145] (1949). The histologic criteria and variations are described in detail. It appears that all the astrocytomas were of the fibrillary type and that none was of the protoplasmatic type. It was found that the malignancy of the majority (52.3 per cent) of the astrocytomas was grade 1; 24.4 per cent were graded 2 in this respect; 17.5 per cent were grade 3; and 5.8 per cent were graded 4. This is in contrast to the malignancy of astrocytomas of the brain, most of which are graded 3 and 4.

In the clinical analysis it was found that astrocytomas occur most frequently in the third to the fifth decade of the patient's life and that males are more often affected than females. Anatomically, astrocytomas were evenly distributed over the spinal cord, in contrast to ependymomas, which exhibited a tendency to develop in the lumbar and sacral segments of the spinal cord and in the filum terminale. The preoperative duration of symptoms manifested a decrease in relation to the increasing histologic malignancy of the lesion, and this duration was 39 months in the case of grade 1 lesions, 29 months in the case of grade 2 lesions, 7 months in the case of grade 3 lesions, and 4 months in the case of grade 4 lesions. Moreover, the postoperative survival rate appeared to be correlated with the histologic grade of malignancy, and decreased from 101 months in the case of grade 1 lesions to 12 months in the case of grade 4 lesions.

Ependymomas also were divided into the four grades of malignancy as indicated by one of us (Kernohan) and associates[145] (1949), and a histologic description of them is given herein. No grade 4 ependymoma, however, was encountered in this series. Sixty-four per cent of all ependymomas were of grade 1 malignancy; 33 per cent, of grade 2 malignancy; and 3 per cent, of grade 3 malignancy. Among the histologic variations of this lesion it appeared that the cellular type was the most common (54.8 per cent), followed by the papillary type (31.7 per cent), mixed type (8.7 per cent), and epithelial type (4.8 per cent). Most of the cellular and epithelial types were found in the spinal cord, whereas the papillary type occurred most frequently in the filum terminale.

The clinical analysis indicates that 50 per cent of ependymomas occur in the fourth and fifth decades of life and that males are more affected than females. In our series the preoperative duration of symptoms of ependymomas of grade 1 was 56 months, and in the case of lesions of grade 2 the preoperative duration was 33 months. Detailed analysis indicates, however, that this difference is less marked in the cellular type of ependymoma of the spinal cord. The postoperative survival of patients who had grade 1 ependymomas averaged 151 months, and among patients who had grade 2 lesions it was 111 months. In this respect, also, the cellular type was found to be exceptional.

Neither among the astrocytomas nor among the ependymomas could a correlation be found between the survival time and the anatomic level at which the tumor of the spinal cord was located.

No suitable basis for the grading of oligodendrogliomas has yet been established. We divided our lesions into oligodendrogliomas and oligodendroblastomas, but the series is too small to permit the formation of any conclusions about this differentiation.

Nongliomatous tumors constituted about 10 per cent of all primary tumors of the spinal cord and filum terminale. They were a diversified group of vascular tumors, lipomas, epidermoids, dermoids, teratomas, neurilemmomas, and a sarcoma. A review of the literature in respect to the concepts of the origin of such lesions is given, and the histologic and clinical details of the cases in question are described.

In Chapter IV abstracts of the clinical histories of the patients are presented in cases in which postmortem examination could be performed. The pathologic findings are described in detail. The relationship between intramedullary tumors of the spinal cord and syringomyelia is discussed. As has been noted previously, there was also in this necropsy series a fairly frequent association of an intramedullary tumor of the spinal cord with syringomyelia (57.6 per cent). This particular association was not restricted to gliomas, but was also found with respect to nongliomatous tumors. The basis of this association remains obscure. In all except one case a close anatomic relationship between both conditions was noted. It was judged that comparison of the structure of the wall of the cavity in cases in which syringomyelia was not associated with an intramedullary tumor with the structure of this wall when syringomyelia was associated with such a lesion disclosed differences in structure which were matters of gradation only. The presence of Rosenthal fibers was, however, rare without the association of syringomyelia with an intramedullary tumor of the spinal cord.

APPENDIX

Salient Data in 301 Cases of Intramedullary Tumors of the Spinal Cord

The data in the 301 cases are presented on pages 194 to 237, which follow.

Reported in Text as Case Number	Age, Years; Sex	Duration, Months			Living or Dead	Symptoms					
		Preop- erative	Postop- erative	Total		Initial	Pain	Sensory Disturb- ance	Motor Disturb- ance	Bladder, Bowel Dys- function	Reflexes, Grade
	Astrocytomas, grade 1
	63 M	18	–	–	Alive, 1960	Pain	Yes	Yes	Yes		Arms, +3
	8 M	84	22	106	Dead	Motor disturbance	No	No	Yes		–3
	45 F	96	336	432	Alive, 1958	Pain	Yes	Yes	Yes		Arms; some di- minished; some ex- aggerated
	27 F	48	72	120	Dead	Pain	Yes	Yes	Yes		Arms, –4
	2 M	15	96	111	Alive, 1960	Motor disturbance	?	?	Yes		Arms, –1
	9 F	1	192	193	Dead	Pain	Yes		Yes		Arms, –4
11	44 F	54	–	–	Dead	Pain	Yes	Yes	Yes		Legs, –3
15	46 M										
	28 F	4	84	88	Alive, 1958	Pain	Yes	No	No		–
	43 F	24	82	106	Alive, 1960	Sensory disturbance	Yes	Yes	Yes		Arms, –2
13	48 F	10	–	–	Dead	Pain	Yes	Yes	Yes		Arms, +1

ntramedullary Tumors of the Spinal Cord

Protein, mg. per 100 cc.	Cells, no. per cu. mm.	Block of Fluid	X-ray Diagnostic for Intraspinal Tumor	Myelogram Diagnostic for Tumor, Spinal Cord	Location According to Vertebral Level	Syringomyelia: Cystic Surgical Lesion, With or Without Histologic Proof	X-ray	Surgical	Comments
					Astrocytomas, grade 1				
55	10		No	Yes	Cervical 1-4		Yes	Biopsy, decompression	
			Yes		Cervical 2-6		Yes	Biopsy, decompression	Papilledema
20	5		No		Cervical 2-7		Yes	Total removal, decompression	
340	6	Yes	No		Cervical 3-5		Yes	Subtotal removal	Re-operation 5 yr. later
750	3		No	Yes	Cervical 3-7			Total removal, decompression	
20	5	Yes	No	Yes	Cervical 3 to thoracic 3	?	Yes	Subtotal removal, decompression	
840	54			Yes	Cervical 3 to thoracic 10	With	Yes	-	
					Cervical 4-6	With		-	Incidental findings
200	1		No	Yes	Cervical 4 to thoracic 2		Yes	Subtotal removal, decompression	Scoliosis
60	1	Yes	No	Yes	Cervical 4 to thoracic 2	With	Yes	Subtotal removal, decompression	
)00	5		No		Cervical 5-6			Biopsy, decompression	Surgical death

Reported in Text as Case Number	Age, Years; Sex	Duration, Months			Living or Dead	Initial	Pain	Sensory Disturbance	Motor Disturbance	Bladder, Bowel Dysfunction	Reflexes, Grade
		Preop-erative	Postop-erative	Total							
	50 M	30	34	64	Dead	Pain	Yes	Yes	Yes		Arms, −4
	34 F	24	48	72	Alive, 1960	Sensory disturbance	No	Yes	Yes		+2
1	21 F	10	21	31	Alive, 1960	Sensory disturbance	No	Yes	Yes		−
2	21 F	84	372	456	?	Motor disturbance	No	Yes	Yes		+
	41 M	108	?	?	?	Pain	Yes	Yes	No		Legs, +2
	25 M	19	156	175	Alive, 1960	Pain	Yes	No	Yes		Arms, −
12	1 4/12 M	13	−	−	Dead	Bladder, bowel dysfunction	Yes	?	Yes	Yes	
	36 M	60	209	269	Dead	Pain	Yes	Yes	Yes		Legs, +1
	29 M	24	194	218	Alive, 1960	Pain	Yes	Yes	No		Legs, +2
	55 M	12	45	57	Dead	Sensory disturbance	No	Yes	Yes		Legs, +3
	43 M	54	24	?	?	Motor disturbance	No	Yes	Yes		Legs, +2
	42 M	144	84	228	Alive, 1960	Motor disturbance	No	Yes	Yes		Legs, +2
	48 M	12	156	168	Alive, 1960	Pain	Yes	Yes	No		Legs, +2
	68 F	66	12	78	Alive, 1960	Motor disturbance	No	Yes	Yes		Legs, +2

Cerebrospinal Fluid			X-ray Diagnostic for Intraspinal Tumor	Myelogram Diagnostic for Tumor, Spinal Cord	Location According to Vertebral Level	Syringomyelia: Cystic Surgical Lesion, With or Without Histologic Proof	Treatment		Comments
Protein, mg. per 100 cc.	Cells, no. per cu. mm.	Block of Fluid					X-ray	Surgical	
					Cervical 5 to thoracic 2	?		Biopsy, decompression	
90	1		No	Yes	Cervical 6 to 7		Yes	Biopsy	Scoliosis
90	2		No	Yes	Cervical 6 to thoracic 1		Yes	Biopsy, decompression	
			No		Cervical 6 to thoracic 3	?		Biopsy, decompression	
			No		Thoracic 1	With		Subtotal removal, decompression	
240	3	Partial block	No		Thoracic 1-3	With	Yes	Subtotal removal	
750	1		No		Thoracic 1-3		-	-	Incidental finding; fibromyxo-sarcoma
500	6	Yes	No		Thoracic 1-4		Yes	Biopsy, decompression	
100	3	Yes		Yes	Thoracic 2	With	Yes	Total removal	
20	1		No	Yes	Thoracic 2-3		Yes	Biopsy, decompression	
20	1		No		Thoracic 2-4	?		Subtotal removal	
50	1		No		Thoracic 2-9	With		Biopsy	
500	6	Partial block	No	Yes	Thoracic 3-4		Yes	Subtotal removal, decompression	
100	1		No	Yes	Thoracic 4-5	With		Subtotal removal	

197

| Reported in Text as Case Number | Age, Years; Sex | Duration, Months | | | Living or Dead | Symptoms | | | | | |
		Preop- erative	Postop- erative	Total		Initial	Pain	Sensory Disturb- ance	Motor Disturb- ance	Bladder, Bowel Dys- function	Reflexes, Grade
	38 M	60	48	108	Dead	Motor disturbance	Yes	Yes	Yes		Legs, +2
	63 M	120	18	138	Alive, 1959	Sensory disturbance	No	Yes	Yes		Legs, +2
	24 F	18	16	34	Dead	Pain	Yes	Yes	Yes		Legs, +2
	20 M	20	20	40	Dead	Pain	Yes	Yes	?	Yes	Legs, +1
	28 F	12	36	?	?	Motor disturbance		Yes	Yes		Legs, +2
14	34 M	96	?	?	Dead	Motor disturbance		Yes	Yes	Yes	Legs, −4
	12 M	1/2	24	?	?	Motor disturbance		?	Yes		Legs, +2
	8 M	78	192	270	Alive, 1960	Motor disturbance		Yes	Yes	Yes	Legs, −2
	29 F	2	36	?	?	Pain	Yes	Yes	Yes		Legs, −4
	36 F	11	120	131	Alive, 1958	Pain	Yes	Yes	No		Legs, −4
	31 F	30	192	222	Alive, 1960	Pain	Yes	No	No	Yes	Legs, +2
	32 F	6	60	?	?	Pain	Yes	Yes	Yes		Legs, −4
	58 M	72	3	75	Dead	Pain	Yes	Yes	Yes		Legs, −4
	39 M	48	312	360	Dead	Pain	Yes	Yes	Yes		Legs, −2
	61 M	12	36	?	?	Sensory disturbance	No	Yes	Yes	Yes	Legs, −3

Cerebrospinal Fluid			X-ray Diagnostic for Intraspinal Tumor	Myelogram Diagnostic for Tumor, Spinal Cord	Location According to Vertebral Level	Syringomyelia: Cystic Surgical Lesion, With or Without Histologic Proof	Treatment		Comments
Protein, mg. per 100 cc.	Cells, no. per cu. mm.	Block of Fluid					X-ray	Surgical	
	13		No		Thoracic 4–8			Total removal, decompression	
45	1		No	Yes	Thoracic 5–7		Yes	Biopsy, decompression	
>1000	5		No		Thoracic 6–8		Yes	Biopsy, decompression	
1600	1	Yes	No	Yes	Thoracic 6–9		Yes	Subtotal removal, decompression	
					Thoracic 7–8		Yes	Total removal	
			No		Thoracic 7 to lumbar 2	With		Biopsy, decompression	Surgical death
200	1		No		Thoracic 9–10	?	Yes	Biopsy, decompression	Scoliosis
2400	1		No		Thoracic 9–11		Yes	Biopsy, decompression	Scoliosis; re-operation 10 yr. later
400	3	Yes	Yes		Thoracic 9–12	?		Subtotal removal, decompression	Scoliosis; calcification
200	6	Partial block	No	Yes	Thoracic 9–12		Yes	Subtotal removal, decompression	
50	2	Partial block		Yes	Thoracic 10–12	?	Yes	Total removal	
3000	5	Yes	Yes	Yes	Thoracic 11	?	Yes	Biopsy, decompression	
	2		No	Yes	Thoracic 11–12		Yes	Subtotal removal	
300	1			Yes	Thoracic 11 to lumbar 1			Biopsy, decompression	
	6		No		Thoracic 11 to lumbar 2			Biopsy, decompression	Scoliosis

199

Reported in Text as Case Number	Age, Years; Sex	Duration, Months			Living or Dead	Symptoms					
		Preop-erative	Postop-erative	Total		Initial	Pain	Sensory Disturb-ance	Motor Disturb-ance	Bladder, Bowel Dys-function	Reflexes, Grade
	22 M	1	96	?	?	Motor disturbance	Yes	Yes	Yes		Legs, −4
	41 M	48	84	132	Alive, 1960	Motor disturbance	No	Yes	No	Yes	Legs, −3
	55 F	4	7	11	Dead	Pain	Yes	Yes	Yes		Legs, −4
	43 F	168	?	?	?	Motor disturbance	Yes	Yes	Yes	Yes	Legs, −4
	25 F	48	276	?	?	Pain	Yes	Yes			Legs, −2
Astrocytomas, grade 2											
	52 M	120	132	252	Dead	Pain	Yes	Yes	Yes		−
	29 M	12	144	?	?	Pain	Yes	Yes	Yes		Legs, +4
	44 F	36	18	54	Dead	Motor disturbance	No	Yes	Yes		Arms, −3
	19 F	2	6	8	Dead	Motor disturbance	Yes	No	Yes		Arms, −2
	34 F	36	6	42	Dead	Pain	Yes	Yes	Yes		
16	21 F	12	−	−	Dead	Pain	Yes	Yes	Yes		Arms, −
	6 M	48	6	?	?	Headache	Yes	No	Yes		Legs, +2
3	67 M	23	16	39	Dead	Pain	Yes	Yes	Yes		Legs, −1
	52 F	108	?	?	?	Motor disturbance	Yes	Yes	Yes		Legs, +3

Cerebrospinal Fluid			X-ray Diagnostic for Intraspinal Tumor	Myelogram Diagnostic for Tumor, Spinal Cord	Location According to Vertebral Level	Syringomyelia: Cystic Surgical Lesion, With or Without Histologic Proof	Treatment		Comments
Protein, mg. per 100 cc.	Cells, no. per cu. mm.	Block of Fluid					X-ray	Surgical	
30	1		No		Thoracic 11 to lumbar 2	?		Biopsy	
150	3	Partial block	No	Yes	Thoracic 12 to lumbar 2	With		Subtotal removal	Conus; re-operation
2000	1		No	Yes	Lumbar 2		Yes	Biopsy, decompression	Conus
			Yes		Lumbar 2			Total removal	Filum
110		Yes	No		Lumbar 2-4			Total removal	Filum
Astrocytomas, grade 2									
60	1		No	Yes	Cervical 1 to thoracic 1	?		Subtotal removal	
600	4	Yes	No		Cervical 2-3			Subtotal removal	
200	5		No		Cervical 3-5		Yes	Biopsy, decompression	
000	60	Partial block	No	Yes	Cervical 4 to thoracic 1			Subtotal removal, decompression	
	6		No		Cervical 5 to thoracic 2			Subtotal removal, decompression	
	5		No		Cervical 6-7			Decompression	Surgical death
300	1		No	Yes	Thoracic 1-3			Subtotal removal, decompression	Neurofibromatosis
300	1		No	Yes	Thoracic 2-3		Yes	Biopsy, decompression	
	1		No		Thoracic 2-3			Biopsy, decompression	

201

Reported in Text as Case Number	Age, Years; Sex	Duration, Months			Living or Dead	Symptoms					
		Preop-erative	Postop-erative	Total		Initial	Pain	Sensory Disturb-ance	Motor Disturb-ance	Bladder, Bowel Dys-function	Reflexes, Grade
	39 M	60	204	?	?	Pain	Yes	Yes	Yes	Yes	Legs, +2
	17 M	2	24	26	Dead	Motor disturbance	No	Yes	Yes		Legs, +4
	48 M	7	30	37	Dead	Pain	Yes	Yes	Yes	Yes	Legs, -4
	61 F	4	120	124	Dead	Pain	Yes	Yes	Yes		Legs, -4
	62 M	36	12	48	Dead	Pain	Yes	Yes	Yes		Legs, -4
	32 M	24	12	36	Dead	Pain	Yes	Yes	Yes		Legs, +1
	57 F	2	11	13	Alive, 1960	Pain	Yes	No	No		Legs, -4
	13 M	3	2	5	Dead	Pain	Yes	No	Yes		Legs, -4
	40 M	36	12	48	Alive, 1959	Pain	Yes	Yes	No		Legs, +3
	23 M	48	324	?	?	Pain	Yes	Yes	No		Legs, +2
	28 F	3	18	21	Dead	Motor disturbance	Yes	Yes	Yes		Legs, -2
	66 M	12	15	27	Dead	Pain	Yes	Yes	Yes		Legs, -2
Astrocytomas, grade 3											
	50 F	10	4	14	Dead	Sensory disturbance	No	Yes	Yes		Legs, +2
	23 F	7	5	12	Dead	Pain	Yes	Yes	Yes		Arms, +1

Cerebrospinal Fluid			X-ray Diagnostic for Intraspinal Tumor	Myelogram Diagnostic for Tumor, Spinal Cord	Location According to Vertebral Level	Syringomyelia: Cystic Surgical Lesion, With or Without Histologic Proof	Treatment		Comments
Protein, mg. per 100 cc.	Cells, no. per cu. mm.	Block of Fluid					X-ray	Surgical	
100	10	Yes	No	Yes	Thoracic 5-10		Yes	Biopsy, decompression	Re-operation 7 yr. later
150	9	Yes	Yes		Thoracic 7			Subtotal removal, decompression	Spina bifida
400	4	Yes	No		Thoracic 7-8	?		Biopsy	
60	1		No	Yes	Thoracic 10			Biopsy, decompression	Scoliosis
			No	Yes	Thoracic 10			Total removal	
360	1	Yes	No	Yes	Thoracic 10-11		Yes	Biopsy, decompression	Surgery 2 yr. before; re-operation 8 mo. after
350	1		No	Yes	Thoracic 10-12		Yes	Biopsy, decompression	
	11	Yes	No	Yes	Thoracic 10-12			Biopsy, decompression	Spina bifida; scoliosis
00	1	Yes	No	No	Thoracic 10-12		Yes	Subtotal removal, decompression	
			No		Thoracic 10 to lumbar 4			Total removal	Filum
30	8	Partial block	No	Yes	Thoracic 12 to lumbar 1		Yes	Subtotal removal	
000		Yes	No		Thoracic 12 to lumbar 1		Yes	Subtotal removal, decompression	
Astrocytomas, grade 3									
90	5	Partial block	No		Cervical 1-3			Subtotal removal, decompression	
00	4		No	Yes	Cervical 1-3			Subtotal removal, decompression	

203

| Reported in Text as Case Number | Age, Years; Sex | Duration, Months | | | Living or Dead | Symptoms | | | | | |
		Preoperative	Postoperative	Total		Initial	Pain	Sensory Disturbance	Motor Disturbance	Bladder, Bowel Dysfunction	Reflexes, Grade
	25 M	4	–	–	Dead	Pain	Yes	Yes	Yes		Arms, –2
	10 F	1	7	8	Dead	Pain	Yes	Yes	Yes		–
	55 F	6	18	24	Dead	Pain	Yes	Yes	Yes		Arms, –4
4	15 F	2	3	5	Dead	Motor disturbance	No	Yes	Yes		Legs, –3
	20 M	4	?	?	?	Motor disturbance		Yes	Yes		Legs, +2
	43 M	1	12	?	?	Sensory disturbance		Yes	Yes		Legs, –4
	38 M	8	12	20	Dead	Pain	Yes	Yes	Yes		Legs, –4
	9 M	13	24	37	Alive, 1959	Pain	Yes	Yes	Yes		Legs, +2
	41 M	12	?	?	?	Pain	Yes	Yes	Yes	Yes	Legs, –4
	32 M	18	56	74	Dead	Pain	Yes	Yes	Yes		Legs, –4
	20 F	11	22	33	Dead	Motor disturbance	Yes	Yes	Yes		Legs, –4
	49 M	8	9	17	Dead	Bladder, bowel dysfunction	Yes	Yes	No	Yes	–
	23 F	6	?	?	?	Pain	Yes	Yes	Yes		Legs, –4

204

Cerebrospinal Fluid			X-ray Diagnostic for Intra-spinal Tumor	Myelogram Diagnostic for Tumor, Spinal Cord	Location According to Vertebral Level	Syringomyelia: Cystic Surgical Lesion, With or Without Histo-logic Proof	Treatment		Comments
Protein, mg. per 100 cc.	Cells, no. per cu. mm.	Block of Fluid					X-ray	Surgical	
	16		No		Cervical 3-4			Biopsy	Papilledema; surgical death
000	2		No	Yes	Cervical 3-5		Yes	Biopsy, decompression	
000	3	Yes	?		Cervical 4-7		Yes	Biopsy, decompression	
		Yes	No		Thoracic 1-3			Subtotal removal, decompression	Scoliosis
			No		Thoracic 2-3			Total removal	
200	3		?		Thoracic 4-7			Subtotal removal, decompression	
500	29			Yes	Thoracic 8 to lumbar 5		Yes	Cordectomy	
50			No		Thoracic 9-12		Yes	Subtotal removal, decompression	Surgery 1 yr. before; re-operation 2 yr. later; scoliosis
		Yes	No		Thoracic 10 to lumbar 2			Biopsy, decompression	
00	2		No	Yes	Thoracic 10 to lumbar ?		Yes	Subtotal removal, decompression	Scoliosis
			No		Thoracic 11 to sacral 1		Yes	Total removal	Filum
00	24		No	?	Thoracic 12 to lumbar 2		Yes	Total removal	Filum
50	35	Yes			Lumbar 3		Yes	Biopsy, decompression	Filum; scoliosis

205

| Reported in Text as Case Number | Age, Years; Sex | Duration, Months | | | Living or Dead | Symptoms | | | | | |
		Preop-erative	Postop-erative	Total		Initial	Pain	Sensory Disturb-ance	Motor Disturb-ance	Bladder, Bowel Dys-function	Reflexes, Grade
						Astrocytomas, grade 4					
	37 F	5	7	12	Dead	Pain	Yes	Yes	Yes		
	7 M	1/2	4	4-1/4	Dead	Motor disturbance	No	No	Yes		Arms, −3
5	27 M	1	36	37	Dead	Sensory disturbance	No	Yes	Yes	Yes	Legs, +4
17	14 F	4	6	10	Dead	Motor disturbance	No	Yes	Yes	Yes	Legs, −3
	32 F	11	7	18	Dead	Motor disturbance	No	Yes	Yes		Legs, −4
						Ependymomas, grade 1					
	51 M	48	180	228	Alive, 1960	Pain	Yes	Yes	Yes		Arms, +1
	36 F	52	48	100	Dead	Pain	Yes	Yes	Yes		Arms, −3
	39 M	84	144	228	?	Motor disturbance	No	Yes	Yes		Legs, +2
	36 M	72	48	120	Alive, 1960	Pain	Yes	Yes	Yes		Arms, −4
	51 F	84	3	87	Dead	Sensory disturbance	Yes	Yes	Yes		Arms, −3
	38 M	10	228	238	Alive, 1960	Motor disturbance	Yes	Yes	Yes		Arms, −4
19	72 F	120?	−	−	Dead	Sensory disturbance					
	44 M	96	2	98	Dead	Sensory disturbance	No	Yes	Yes		Arms, −3
	65 M	240	120	360	Dead	Pain	Yes	Yes	?		Arms, −2

Cerebrospinal Fluid			X-ray Diagnostic for Intraspinal Tumor	Myelogram Diagnostic for Tumor, Spinal Cord	Location According to Vertebral Level	Syringomyelia: Cystic Surgical Lesion, With or Without Histologic Proof	Treatment		Comments
Protein, mg. per 100 cc.	Cells, no. per cu. mm.	Block of Fluid					X-ray	Surgical	
Astrocytomas, grade 4									
				Yes	Cervical 1-5		Yes	Subtotal removal, decompression	
600	29	Yes	No		Cervical 6 to thoracic 1		Yes	Total removal	
					Cervical 7 to lumbar 5		Yes	Cordectomy	Surgery, x-ray treatment before coming to clinic
			No		Thoracic 7-8		Yes	Decompression	
			No		Thoracic 8			Biopsy	
Ependymomas, grade 1									
20	1		No		Cervical 1-4	?	-	Subtotal removal	
	10	Partial block	No		Cervical 1 to thoracic 1	?	Yes	Subtotal removal, decompression	
50	4	Yes	No		Cervical 2-3		Yes	Subtotal removal	
300	12		No	Yes	Cervical 2-3	?	Yes	Biopsy, decompression	Scoliosis; spina bifida
60	4		No		Cervical 2-7	?		Subtotal removal	
60	5	Partial block	No		Cervical 3-6			Subtotal removal, decompression	Carcinoma, rectum
					Cervical 3			-	Incidental finding
20	2	Yes	Yes?		Cervical 4-7	?	Yes	Subtotal removal, decompression	
90	2	Partial block			Cervical 4-7		Yes	Subtotal removal, decompression	Re-operation 6 yr. later

207

Reported in Text as Case Number	Age, Years; Sex	Duration, Months			Living or Dead	Symptoms					
		Preoperative	Postoperative	Total		Initial	Pain	Sensory Disturbance	Motor Disturbance	Bladder, Bowel Dysfunction	Reflexes, Grade
	55 M	120	–	–	Dead	Sensory disturbance	No	Yes	Yes		Arms, +1
	54 F	64	120	184	Alive, 1960	Pain	Yes	Yes	Yes		Arms, -1
	39 M	96	144	240	Alive, 1960	Motor disturbance	No	Yes	Yes		Arms, -3
	31 M	24	216	240	Alive, 1960	Pain	Yes	Yes	Yes		Arms, -1
	41 F	–	24		Alive, 1960	?	No	Yes	Yes		Legs, +3
	35 M	72	36	108	Alive, 1960	Sensory disturbance	Yes	Yes	Yes	Yes	Legs, +3
20	46 M	11	2	13	Dead	Pain	Yes	Yes	Yes		Legs, -4
	50 F	15	36	51	Dead	Pain	Yes	Yes	?		Legs, +1
	57 M	60	–	–	?	Motor disturbance	Yes	Yes	Yes	Yes	Legs, +4
	37 M	12	84	96	Dead	Pain	Yes	Yes	Yes		Legs, +3
21	52 M	120	–	–	Dead	Bladder, bowel dysfunction	No	Yes	Yes	Yes	Legs, +4
	41 M	26	40	66	Dead	Pain	Yes	Yes	Yes		Legs, +3
	48 M	9	57	66	Dead	Sensory disturbance	No	Yes	Yes	Yes	Arms, -4
	53 M	28	18	46	Dead	Pain	Yes	Yes	Yes	Yes	?

Intramedullary Tumors of the Spinal Cord (Continued)

Cerebrospinal Fluid			X-ray Diagnostic for Intra- spinal Tumor	Myelogram Diagnostic for Tumor, Spinal Cord	Location According to Vertebral Level	Syringomyelia: Cystic Surgical Lesion, With or Without Histo- logic Proof	Treatment		Comments
Protein, mg. per 100 cc.	Cells, no. per cu. mm.	Block of Fluid					X-ray	Surgical	
200	1		No		Cervical 4 to thoracic 1			Total removal	Surgical death
20	2			Yes	Cervical 5-7	?	–	Subtotal removal	
85	3	Yes	No		Cervical 6 to thoracic 1	With	Yes	Subtotal removal, decompression	
95	1		No		Cervical 6 to thoracic 1	?	Yes	Subtotal removal	
1000	1		No	Yes	Cervical 6 to thoracic 8			Subtotal removal	
1000	1	Yes	No	Yes	Cervical 6 to thoracic 8		Yes	Total removal	
	18		No		Thoracic 1-3	With		Biopsy, decompression	Surgical death
100	1		Yes	Yes	Thoracic 1-4			Subtotal removal, decompression	
			No		Thoracic 1-4	?	Yes	Biopsy	
			No		Thoracic 1-4			Biopsy, decompression	
400	14		No		Thoracic 1-4	With	–	Total removal	Surgical death; subependy- mal glioma at thoracic 9
					Thoracic 1-5		Yes	Subtotal removal	
			No		Thoracic 1-?			Biopsy, decompression	
		Yes		Yes	Thoracic 2-4	With	Yes	Biopsy, decompression	

209

| Reported in Text as Case Number | Age, Years; Sex | Duration, Months | | | Living or Dead | Initial | Symptoms | | | | Reflexes, Grade |
		Preop-erative	Postop-erative	Total			Pain	Sensory Disturb-ance	Motor Disturb-ance	Bladder, Bowel Dys-function	
6	35 M	36	120	156	Alive, 1960	Pain	Yes	Yes	?		Legs, +2
	41 F	24	168	192	?	Sensory disturbance	No	Yes	Yes		Legs, +3
	31 M	18	96	114	Dead	Sensory disturbance	Yes	Yes	Yes	Yes	Legs, +3
	52 F	21	276	297	Dead	Motor disturbance	Yes	Yes	Yes	Yes	Legs, +1
	50 M	39	96	135	Alive, 1960	Sensory disturbance	Yes	Yes	Yes		Legs, +2
	51 M	72	348	420	Dead	Motor disturbance	Yes	Yes	Yes	Yes	Legs, +3
22	46 M	120	–	–	Dead	Sensory disturbance	No	Yes	Yes		Legs, +2
	22 F	22	108	130	Dead	Pain	Yes	Yes	Yes	Yes	Legs, -4
	33 F	36	36	72	Dead	Motor disturbance	Yes	Yes	Yes		Legs, -4
	41 M	16	204	220	Alive, 1960	Sensory disturbance	Yes	Yes	Yes		Legs, +1
	29 M	72	348	420	?	Pain	Yes	Yes	Yes		Legs, -3
	36 F	26	204	230	Dead	Pain	Yes	Yes	Yes		Legs, +1 -3
	26 F	16	48	64	Dead	Pain	Yes	Yes	Yes		Legs, -4
	32 M	48	216	264	Alive, 1960	Pain	Yes	Yes	Yes	Yes	Legs, +2

Cerebrospinal Fluid			X-ray Diagnostic for Intraspinal Tumor	Myelogram Diagnostic for Tumor, Spinal Cord	Location According to Vertebral Level	Syringomyelia: Cystic Surgical Lesion, With or Without Histologic Proof	Treatment		Comments
Protein, mg. per 100 cc.	Cells, no. per cu. mm.	Block of Fluid					X-ray	Surgical	
25	1	Partial block	No	Yes	Thoracic 2-4	With	Yes	Total removal	
			No		Thoracic 3-6	?		Subtotal removal, decompression	
360	10	Yes	No		Thoracic 4-6	With	Yes	Subtotal removal, decompression	
	2		No		Thoracic 4-6	?		Biopsy, decompression	
95	1		No	Yes	Thoracic 4-7	?	Yes	Subtotal removal, decompression	
	6	Partial block	No		Thoracic 7-9	With		Biopsy, decompression	
					Thoracic 7-11	With		Subtotal removal	Spina bifida; surgical death
			No	Yes	Thoracic 8-10	?		Subtotal removal	
4000		Yes	No		Thoracic 8-11		Yes	Biopsy, decompression	
300	3	Yes	No		Thoracic 8-?		Yes	Subtotal removal, decompression	
Dry		Yes	No		Thoracic 8 to lumbar 2		Yes	Subtotal removal	Filum
640	7		No		Thoracic 9 to lumbar 1	?	Yes	Subtotal removal, decompression	Re-operation 6 yr. later
		Yes	No		Thoracic 9 to lumbar 2			Subtotal removal, decompression	Conus, filum
		Yes	Yes		Thoracic 9 to lumbar 3		Yes	Subtotal removal, decompression	Conus, filum

Reported in Text as Case Number	Age, Years; Sex	Duration, Months			Living or Dead	Symptoms					
		Preop-erative	Postop-erative	Total		Initial	Pain	Sensory Disturb-ance	Motor Disturb-ance	Bladder, Bowel Dys-function	Reflexes, Grade
	43 F	144	228	372	Dead	Pain	Yes	Yes	No		Legs, −4
	32 M	96	−	−	?	Pain	Yes	Yes	Yes	Yes	Legs, −2
	10 F	18	36	54	Alive, 1959	Pain	Yes	No	Yes		Legs, −4
	49 F	180	48	228	Dead	Sensory disturbance	Yes	Yes	Yes		Legs, −4
	17 F	96	132	228	Alive, 1960	Pain	Yes	Yes	Yes		Legs, −4
	33 M	48	432	480	Alive, 1960	Pain	Yes	No	Yes		−
	32 M	96	8	104	Dead	Pain	Yes	Yes	Yes		Legs, −4
	50 F	24	60	84	Alive, 1960	Sensory disturbance	No	Yes	No		Legs, −2
	43 M	120	132	252	Alive, 1960	Motor disturbance	No	Yes	Yes	Yes	Legs, −4
	36 M	12	240	252	Alive, 1960	Pain	Yes	No	No		Legs, +1
	34 M	108	180	288	?	Pain	Yes	Yes	Yes	Yes	Legs, −4
23	26 M	60	−	−	Dead	Pain	Yes	Yes	Yes		Legs, −2

212

Cerebrospinal Fluid			X-ray Diagnostic for Intra-spinal Tumor	Myelogram Diagnostic for Tumor, Spinal Cord	Location According to Vertebral Level	Syringomyelia: Cystic Surgical Lesion, With or Without Histo-logic Proof	Treatment		Comments
Protein, mg. per 100 cc.	Cells, no. per cu. mm.	Block of Fluid					X-ray	Surgical	
		Yes	No		Thoracic 9 to lumbar 3		Yes	Biopsy, decompression	Conus, filum, papilledema
		Yes	No		Thoracic 9 to lumbar 4		Yes	Subtotal removal	Filum; spondy-lolisthesis
Dry			No		Thoracic 9 to sacral 1		Yes	Subtotal removal, decompression	Scoliosis
Dry			No		Thoracic 10 to lumbar 4		Yes	Subtotal removal	Carcinoma, uterus
Dry			Yes		Thoracic 10 to lumbar 4		Yes	Total removal	Kyphoscolio-sis; re-operation
Dry			No		Thoracic 10 to lumbar 5		Yes	Total removal	
			No		Thoracic 10 to lumbar 5			Subtotal removal, decompression	
200	1		No	Yes	Thoracic 11 to lumbar 1		Yes	Subtotal removal	
120	1		No	Yes	Thoracic 11 to lumbar 1			Total removal	Spina bitida
000	30	Yes	No	?	Thoracic 11 to lumbar 1			Total removal	
			No		Thoracic 11 to lumbar 1			Total removal	Conus, filum
			No		Thoracic 11 to lumbar 2			Biopsy	Spina bifida; surgical death

213

Reported in Text as Case Number	Age, Years; Sex	Duration, Months			Living or Dead	Symptoms					Reflexes, Grade
		Preop- erative	Postop- erative	Total		Initial	Pain	Sensory Disturb- ance	Motor Disturb- ance	Bladder, Bowel Dys- function	
	50 M	96	144	240	Alive, 1960	Motor disturbance	Yes	Yes	Yes		Legs, −3
7	12 M	12	132	144	Alive, 1960	Pain	Yes	No	Yes		Legs +1
	35 M	60	372	432	Dead	Pain	Yes	Yes	Yes	Yes	Legs, −3
	52 M	204	144	346	Alive, 1960	Pain	Yes	Yes	No	Yes	Legs, +1
	36 F	15	48	63	Dead	Pain	Yes	Yes	Yes	Yes	Legs, −4
	6 M	7	12	19	Alive, 1959	Pain	Yes	No	?	Yes	Legs, +3
	27 F	48	360	408	Dead	Pain	Yes	Yes	Yes		Legs, −4
	28 F	24	–	–	Dead	Pain	Yes	Yes	Yes		Legs, −4
	26 M	120	408	528	Alive, 1960	Pain	Yes	Yes	Yes	Yes	Legs, −3
	30 M	19	168	187	Alive, 1960	Pain	Yes	No	No		
	33 M	18	252	270	Alive, 1959	Pain	Yes	Yes	No		Legs, −3
	30 F	48	132	180	Alive, 1960	Pain	Yes	No	No	Yes	Legs, −1
	27 F	22	252	274	Alive, 1960	Pain	Yes	No	No		Legs, +1

Cerebrospinal Fluid			X-ray Diagnostic for Intra-spinal Tumor	Myelogram Diagnostic for Tumor, Spinal Cord	Location According to Vertebral Level	Syringomyelia: Cystic Surgical Lesion, With or Without Histo-logic Proof	Treatment		Comments
Protein, mg. per 100 cc.	Cells, no. per cu. mm.	Block of Fluid					X-ray	Surgical	
4000		Yes	No		Thoracic 11 to lumbar 3			Total removal	Wedging, thoracic 12
180	1		Yes		Thoracic 11 to lumbar 3			Total removal	Papilledema
			No		Thoracic 11 to lumbar 3			Total removal	
0,000	1	Yes	No	Yes	Thoracic 11 to lumbar 3		Yes	Total removal	
			No		Thoracic 11 to lumbar 4			Subtotal removal, decompression	Conus, filum
’500	16		No	Yes	Thoracic 11 to lumbar 4		Yes	Total removal	
			No		Thoracic 11 to lumbar 4			Total removal	Conus, filum
			No		Thoracic 11 to lumbar 5			Subtotal removal	Surgical death
			No		Thoracic 11 to lumbar 5			Total removal	Scoliosis
000			No	Yes	Thoracic 12 to lumbar 1			Total removal	
600			No	Yes	Thoracic 12 to lumbar 1			Total removal	
			No		Thoracic 12 to lumbar 1			Total removal	Scoliosis
900	2	Par-tial block	No	Yes	Thoracic 12 to lumbar 2		Yes	Total removal	

Reported in Text as Case Number	Age, Years; Sex	Duration, Months			Living or Dead	Symptoms					
		Preop- erative	Postop- erative	Total		Initial	Pain	Sensory Disturb- ance	Motor Disturb- ance	Bladder, Bowel Dys- function	Reflexes, Grade
	33 M	30	84	114	Alive, 1960	Pain	Yes	Yes	No	Yes	Legs, −3
	53 M	24	216	240	Alive, 1960	Pain	Yes	No	No		Legs, −4
	34 M	24	168	192	Alive 1960	Pain	Yes	No	No		Legs, +1
	55 M	36	96	132	Dead	Pain	Yes	Yes	Yes	Yes	Legs, −4
	32 F	24	204	228	Alive, 1959	Pain	Yes	No	No		Legs, −1
	18 F	22	120	142	Alive, 1960	Pain	Yes	Yes	Yes	Yes	Legs, −4
	29 M	40	−	−	Dead	Pain	Yes	No	No		Legs, −2
	48 M	24	264	288	Alive, 1960	Pain	Yes	Yes	Yes		Legs, −3
	34 M	108	144	252	Alive, 1960	Pain	Yes	Yes	Yes		Legs
	21 F	36	132	168	?	Pain	Yes	No	No		Legs, −3
	43 F	2	144	146	Alive, 1960	Pain	Yes	No	No		Legs, +1
	29 M	9	144	153	Alive, 1960	Pain	Yes	Yes	Yes		Legs, −
	12 M	5	24	29	Alive, 1958	Pain	Yes	No	No		−
	46 M	48	144	192	?	Pain	Yes	No	Yes		Legs, −4
	82 F	30	12	42	Alive, 1960	Pain	Yes	No	No	Yes	Legs ?

Cerebrospinal Fluid			X-ray Diagnostic for Intra-spinal Tumor	Myelogram Diagnostic for Tumor, Spinal Cord	Location According to Vertebral Level	Syringomyelia: Cystic Surgical Lesion, With or Without Histo-logic Proof	Treatment		Comments
Protein, mg. per 100 cc.	Cells, no. per cu. mm.	Block of Fluid					X-ray	Surgical	
700	3	Partial block	No		Thoracic 12 to lumbar 3		Yes	Biopsy, decompression	
350	3	Yes	No	Yes	Thoracic 12 to lumbar 3		Yes	Total removal	Lumbosacral anomaly
5000	5	Partial block	No	Yes	Thoracic 12 to lumbar 3			Total removal	
9000	0	Yes	No	Yes	Thoracic 12 to lumbar 3			Subtotal removal	
			No	Yes	Thoracic 12 to lumbar 4			Subtotal removal	
8000	2		No	Yes	Thoracic 12 to lumbar 4			Subtotal removal	
	3	Yes	No		Thoracic 12 to lumbar 5		Yes	Total removal	Sacraliza-tion lumbar 5
4000	3	Yes	No		Thoracic 12 to lumbar 5			Subtotal removal	Syphilis
240	3	Partial block		Yes	Lumbar 1-2			Total removal	
8000			Yes		Lumbar 1-2		Yes	Total removal	
3000		Yes	Yes	Yes	Lumbar 1-3		Yes	Total removal	
8000	2		No	Yes	Lumbar 1-3		Yes	Total removal	
100	10		No	Yes	Lumbar 1-4		Yes	Total removal	
8000			No	Yes?	Lumbar 1-4			Total removal	
0,000			No	?	Lumbar 1-4			Subtotal removal	Scoliosis

217

Reported in Text as Case Number	Age, Years; Sex	Duration, Months			Living or Dead	Symptoms					
		Preop-erative	Postop-erative	Total		Initial	Pain	Sensory Disturb-ance	Motor Disturb-ance	Bladder, Bowel Dys-function	Reflexes, Grade
	39 M	7	204	211	Alive, 1960	Pain	Yes	No	No		Legs, +1
	14 M	12	204	216	Alive, 1960	Pain	Yes	No	No		Legs, -2
25	51 M	-	-	-	Dead						
	32 F	40	204	244	Alive, 1960	Pain	Yes	No	No		Legs, -2
	26 F	36	-	-	?	Pain	Yes	No	No		Legs, +1
	39 F	96	24	120	Dead	Pain	Yes	Yes	Yes		Legs, -4
	46 F	180	192	372	Alive, 1960	Pain	Yes	Yes	Yes		Legs, -3
	33 F	120	276	396	Alive, 1960	Pain	Yes	No	No		?
	31 F	36	216	252	?	Pain	Yes	No	No		Legs, +1
	18 F	29	192	221	Alive, 1960	Pain	Yes	No	No		Legs, +1
	22 M	15	156	171	Dead	Pain	Yes	No	Yes		-
	28 F	36	24	60	Dead	Pain	Yes	No	No		Legs, +1
	19 M	10	252	262	Alive, 1960	Pain	Yes	No	No		-
	49 M	72	240	312	Alive, 1960	Pain	Yes	No	Yes		Legs, -1
	35 F	18	384	402	Alive, 1960	Pain	Yes	Yes	Yes		Legs, +1
	44 M	54	2	56	Dead	Pain	Yes	No	No		
	36 M	32	108	140	?	Pain	Yes	No	No		Legs, -1

Cerebrospinal Fluid			X-ray Diagnostic for Intra-spinal Tumor	Myelogram Diagnostic for Tumor, Spinal Cord	Location According to Vertebral Level	Syringomyelia: Cystic Surgical Lesion, With or Without Histo-logic Proof	Treatment		Comments
Protein, mg. per 100 cc.	Cells, no. per cu. mm.	Block of Fluid					X-ray	Surgical	
7000		Yes	No		Lumbar 1-5			Total removal	
280	12	Yes	No		Lumbar 1-5			Total removal	Spondylolis-thesis
					Filum			–	Incidental finding
5500		Yes	No	Yes	Lumbar 1-5			Total removal	
1200			No	No	Lumbar 1-5			Total removal	
Dry			No		Lumbar 1-5			Subtotal removal	
			Yes		Lumbar to sacral			Total removal	
120		Yes	No		Lumbar 2-3			Total removal	
450	2	Yes	Yes	Yes	Lumbar 2-3			Total removal	Spina bifida
250	1	Yes	No	Yes	Lumbar 2-4			Total removal	
600	5		No		Lumbar 2-4			Total removal	Died, tuber-culosis
140	4		No	Yes	Lumbar 2-4			Total removal	Died, ileus
800	31	Yes	No		Lumbar 2-4			Total removal	Scoliosis
			Yes		Lumbar 2-5		Yes	Total removal	
			No		Lumbar 2-5			Total removal	
2500	27	Yes	Yes	No	Lumbar 3			Total removal	Died, syphilitic meningitis
			No		Lumbar 3-4			Total removal	

Reported in Text as Case Number	Age, Years; Sex	Duration, Months			Living or Dead	Symptoms					
		Preop-erative	Postop-erative	Total		Initial	Pain	Sensory Disturb-ance	Motor Disturb-ance	Bladder, Bowel Dys-function	Reflexes, Grade
	61 M	16	96	112	Alive, 1960	Pain	Yes	No	No		Legs, −1
	55 F	180	96	276	Alive, 1960	Pain	Yes	Yes	Yes		Legs, +1
24	23 F	60	−	−	Dead	Pain	Yes	Yes	Yes		Legs, −4
	21 F	36	108	144	?	Pain	Yes	No	No		−
	47 M	16	120	136	Dead	Pain	Yes	No	No		?
	46 F	24	96	120	?	Pain	Yes	No	No		−
	37 M	72	192	?	Dead	Pain	Yes	Yes	No	Yes	
26	62 F	−	−	−	Dead						
	29 F	30	168	198	Alive, 1960	Pain	Yes	No	No		−
	28 M	48	240	288	Alive, 1960	Pain	Yes	No	Yes		Legs, −3
	46 M	120	24	144	Alive, 1960	Pain	Yes	Yes	No		Legs, +1
	36 M	144	132	276	Dead	Pain	Yes	Yes	No		Legs, +1
	32 M	144	420	564	Alive, 1960	Pain	Yes	Yes	No		Legs, −4
	19 M	9	276	285	Alive, 1960	Pain	Yes	Yes	Yes		Legs, −1

Cerebrospinal Fluid			X-ray Diagnostic for Intraspinal Tumor	Myelogram Diagnostic for Tumor, Spinal Cord	Location According to Vertebral Level	Syringomyelia: Cystic Surgical Lesion, With or Without Histologic Proof	Treatment		Comments
Protein, mg. per 100 cc.	Cells, no. per cu. mm.	Block of Fluid					X-ray	Surgical	
500	3		No		Lumbar 3-4			Total removal	
			Yes		Lumbar 3-5		Yes	Subtotal removal, decompression	
					Lumbar 3-5	With		Subtotal removal	Surgical death
3800	1		No	Yes	Lumbar 3-5		Yes	Subtotal removal	
50	4		No		Lumbar 3 to sacral 1		Yes	Total removal	Spina bifida occulta
			No	Yes	Lumbar 3 to sacral 1			Total removal	Sacralization, lumbar 5
	9		Yes		Lumbar 3 to sacral 3			Total removal	
					Filum				Incidental finding
Dry		Yes	No	Yes	Lumbar 4		Yes	Total removal	
Dry		Yes	No	Yes	Lumbar 4-5		Yes	Subtotal removal	Re-operation 14 yr. later
200	1		No		Lumbar 4 to sacral 2		Yes	Subtotal removal	
40	2		Yes	Yes	Lumbar 4 to sacral 3			Subtotal removal	
			No		Sacral 1-3		Yes	Subtotal removal	Spina bifida; carcinoma, bladder
					Sacrum		Yes	Subtotal removal	

Reported in Text as Case Number	Age, Years; Sex	Duration, Months			Living or Dead	Symptoms					
		Preop-erative	Postop-erative	Total		Initial	Pain	Sensory Disturb-ance	Motor Disturb-ance	Bladder, Bowel Dys-function	Reflexes, Grade
						Ependymomas, grade 2					
	54 F	48	96	144	Alive, 1959	Sensory disturbance	Yes	Yes	?		Legs, +2
	35 M	36	144	180	Alive, 1960	Motor disturbance	No	Yes	Yes		Arms, +2
	40 M	48	276	328	Dead	Motor disturbance	No	Yes	Yes		
	57 F	5	–	–	?	Pain	Yes	Yes	Yes		Arms, –4
	21 F	72	21	93	Dead	Motor disturbance	No	Yes	Yes		Arms, –4
27	62 M	–	–	–	Dead						
28	40 M	13	–	–	Dead						
	40 F	84	–	–	?	Sensory disturbance	Yes	Yes	Yes		Arms, –2
8	42 M	108	48	156	Alive, 1960	Pain	Yes	Yes	No	Yes	Arms, +−
	38 F	18	276	294	Alive, 1960	Pain	Yes	Yes	Yes		Arms, –3
	42 M	42	84	126	Alive, 1960	Sensory disturbance	No	Yes	Yes		Arms, –3
	49 M	72	108	180	Alive, 1960	Pain	Yes	Yes	Yes		Arms, –4
	42 F	48	12	60	Alive, 1959	Pain	Yes	Yes	Yes	Yes	Arms, –2
29	44 M	24	36	60	Dead	Pain	Yes	Yes	Yes		Arms, –3

Cerebrospinal Fluid			X-ray Diagnostic for Intra-spinal Tumor	Myelogram Diagnostic for Tumor, Spinal Cord	Location According to Vertebral Level	Syringomyelia: Cystic Surgical Lesion, With or Without Histologic Proof	Treatment		Comments
Protein, mg. per 100 cc.	Cells, no. per cu. mm.	Block of Fluid					X-ray	Surgical	
Ependymomas, grade 2									
			No		Occiput to cervical 3		Yes	Subtotal removal, decompression	Multiple neuro-fibromas
140	1	Yes	No		Cervical 1-2	With	Yes	Subtotal removal, decompression	
80	3	Par-tial block	?		Cervical 2-6			Total removal	Carcinoma, testis and rectum
100	2		No		Cervical 2-7			Subtotal removal	
			No		Cervical 2 to thoracic 2			Biopsy, decompression	
					Cervical 3-4				Incidental finding
					Cervical 4				Incidental finding
40	2		No	Yes	Cervical 4-7	?	Yes	Decompression	Re-operation 3 yr. later
160	2	Yes	No	Yes	Cervical 4 to thoracic 4		Yes	Subtotal removal, decompression	
200	4	Yes	?		Cervical 5-6	?	Yes	Subtotal removal, decompression	
75	1		No		Cervical 5-6		Yes	Subtotal removal	
400	17	Yes	No		Cervical 5-7			Subtotal removal, decompression	
100	1	Par-tial block	No	Yes	Cervical 5-7		Yes	Subtotal removal, decompression	
000		Yes	Yes		Cervical 5-7	With	Yes	Subtotal removal	Died after re-operation

Reported in Text as Case Number	Age, Years; Sex	Duration, Months			Living or Dead	Symptoms					Reflexes, Grade
		Preop- erative	Postop- erative	Total		Initial	Pain	Sensory Disturb- ance	Motor Disturb- ance	Bladder, Bowel Dys- function	
	33 M	18	240	258	Alive, 1960	Sensory disturbance	No	Yes	Yes	Yes	?
	35 F	36	192	228	Alive, 1960	Bladder, bowel dysfunction	No	Yes	Yes	Yes	Legs, +4
30	37 F	18	–	–	Dead	Sensory disturbance	No	Yes	No		Legs, +2
	35 M	72	24	96	Dead	Motor disturbance	No	Yes	Yes	Yes	Legs, +3
	16 F	6	84	90	Dead	Pain	Yes	Yes	Yes		Legs, –4
	37 M	48	24	72	Alive, 1960	Sensory disturbance	No	Yes	Yes		Legs, –1
	48 M	36	144	180	Dead	Pain	Yes	No	No		
	28 F	24	300	324	Alive, 1960	Pain	Yes	No	?		Legs, –4
	43 M	60	–	–	?	Sensory disturbance	Yes	Yes	Yes	Yes	Legs, +2
	53 M	204	96	300	Dead	Sensory disturbance	Yes	Yes	Yes		Legs, +4
	45 F	12	24	36	Dead	Motor disturbance	Yes	Yes	Yes	Yes	Legs, +4
	54 F	72	84	156	Dead	Motor disturbance	No	Yes	Yes	Yes	Legs, +3
	16 F	8	108	116	Alive, 1960	Pain	Yes	No	No		–
	17 M	3	–	–	Dead	Bladder, bowel dysfunction	No	Yes	Yes	Yes	Legs, –4
	28 F	48	216	264	Alive, 1960	Pain	Yes	Yes	Yes	Yes	Legs, –2

Cerebrospinal Fluid			X-ray Diagnostic for Intraspinal Tumor	Myelogram Diagnostic for Tumor, Spinal Cord	Location According to Vertebral Level	Syringomyelia: Cystic Surgical Lesion, With or Without Histologic Proof	Treatment		Comments
Protein, mg. per 100 cc.	Cells, no. per cu. mm.	Block of Fluid					X-ray	Surgical	
300	8	Yes	No		Cervical 6-7			Total removal	
1000	6	Yes	No		Cervical 7 to thoracic 2		Yes	Subtotal removal	
100	1		No	Yes	Cervical 7 to thoracic 2	With	No	Subtotal removal	Surgical death
			No		Cervical 7 to thoracic 4	With		?	
320	5	Yes	No	Yes	Thoracic 1-5		Yes	Subtotal removal, decompression	Neuro-fibroma, thigh
150	1		No	Yes	Thoracic 3-6	With	Yes	Biopsy, decompression	
1600	9	Yes	No		Thoracic 4-6			Subtotal, removal, decompression	
160	3	Yes	No	Yes	Thoracic 5-10	With	Yes	Total removal	Re-operation
			No		Thoracic 6-9	With		Total removal	
					Thoracic 8-9			Subtotal removal	Died, cerebral hemorrhage
40	2		No		Thoracic 8-10			Biopsy	
88			No		Thoracic 8-12			Total removal	Scoliosis
500	1	Par- tial block	No	Yes	Thoracic 10 to lumbar 3		Yes	Total removal	Scoliosis
			Yes		Thoracic 10 to lumbar 5			Total removal	
450	5		No	Yes	Thoracic 11 to lumbar 1	?	Yes	Subtotal removal	Lumbosacral anomaly

Reported in Text as Case Number	Age, Years; Sex	Duration, Months			Living or Dead	Symptoms					
		Preop-erative	Postop-erative	Total		Initial	Pain	Sensory Disturb-ance	Motor Disturb-ance	Bladder, Bowel Dys-function	Reflexes, Grade
	35 F	5	12	17	Dead	Pain	Yes	Yes	Yes	Yes	Legs, -4
	35 F	18	240	258	Alive, 1960	Pain	Yes	No	No		Legs, +1
	46 M	36	24	60	Alive, 1960	Motor disturbance	No	No	Yes		Legs, -4
	22 F	36	108	144	Alive, 1960	Pain	Yes	Yes	Yes		Legs, -3
	18 F	12	108	120	?	Pain	Yes	No	No		-
	25 F	12	264	276	Alive, 1960	Pain	Yes	Yes	Yes		Legs, -4
31	33 M	18	22	40	Dead	Impotence	Yes	Yes	Yes		Legs, -3
	23 F	48	204	252	Alive, 1960	Pain	Yes	No	No		-
	40 M	39	44	83	Alive, 1960	Pain	Yes	No	Yes		Legs, -2
	21 F	42	36	78	Dead	Pain	Yes	Yes	Yes		Legs, -4
	41 M	16	180	196	Dead	Pain	Yes	No	No		-
	50 M	6	252	258	Dead	Pain	Yes	No	No		-
	57 M	12	24	36	Alive, 1960	Pain	Yes	Yes	Yes		Legs, -4
	58 M	?	156	?	Alive, 1960	Pain	Yes	Yes	No		Legs, -3
	30 F	15	9	24	Dead	Pain	Yes	Yes	No		Legs, +2

Intramedullary Tumors of the Spinal Cord (Continued)

Cerebrospinal Fluid			X-ray Diagnostic for Intra-spinal Tumor	Myelogram Diagnostic for Tumor, Spinal Cord	Location According to Vertebral Level	Syringomyelia: Cystic Surgical Lesion, With or Without Histo-logic Proof	Treatment		Comments
Protein, mg. per 100 cc.	Cells, no. per cu. mm.	Block of Fluid					X-ray	Surgical	
10,000	1	Yes	No	Yes	Thoracic 11 to lumbar 3		Yes	Subtotal removal, decompression	
4000			No		Thoracic 12 to lumbar 2		Yes	Total removal	
100	1		No	Yes	Thoracic 12 to lumbar 2		Yes	Total removal	
120	5	Yes	Yes		Thoracic 12 to lumbar 3		Yes	Total removal	Gross calcification tumor
8000			No	Yes	Thoracic 12 to lumbar 4			Total removal	
			No		Thoracic 12 to lumbar 4			Total removal	
600	8		Yes	Yes	Thoracic 12 to lumbar 5			Total removal	Recurrence
6000		Yes	No	Yes	Lumbar 1-3			Subtotal removal	
300	1		No	Yes	Lumbar 1-3		Yes	Subtotal removal	Papilledema
Dry		Yes	No		Lumbar 1-5			Subtotal removal	
500		Yes	No	Yes	Lumbar 2-4			Total removal	Re-operation 9 yr. later
2400		Yes	No		Lumbar 2-4			Total removal	Re-operation 13 yr. later
450	2		No	?	Lumbar 2-4			Subtotal removal, decompression	Four lumbar vertebrae
600					Lumbar 2-?			Subtotal removal	
750	17		Yes		Lumbar 2-5		Yes	Subtotal removal, decompression	

227

Reported in Text as Case Number	Age, Years; Sex	Duration, Months			Living or Dead	Symptoms					
		Preoperative	Postoperative	Total		Initial	Pain	Sensory Disturbance	Motor Disturbance	Bladder, Bowel Dysfunction	Reflexes, Grade
	33 M	10	–	–	?	Pain	Yes	No	Yes		Legs, +1
	48 F	4	108	112	Alive, 1960	Pain	Yes	No	?		Legs, +1
	59 M	3	15	18	Alive, 1960	Pain	Yes	No	No		–
	22 F	60	228	288	Alive, 1960	Pain	Yes	Yes	No		Legs, +1
	25 F	17	–	–	?	Pain	Yes	No	?		
	32 M	6	156	162	Alive, 1960	Pain	Yes	No	No		Legs, +1
	56 M	8	30	38	Dead	Bladder, bowel dysfunction	No	Yes	Yes	Yes	Legs, –4
	14 M	24	33	57	Dead	Pain	Yes	Yes	Yes	Yes	Legs, –4
	57 M	15	–	–	?	Pain	Yes	Yes	No	Yes	Legs, –2
	64 M	2	12	14	Dead	Pain	Yes	No	No		–
	18 M	7	60	67	Dead	Pain	Yes	No	?		–
9	14 M	15	144	159	Dead	Pain	Yes	Yes	Yes	Yes	–
Ependymomas, grade 3											
	61 F	7	38	45	Dead	Sensory disturbance	No	Yes	Yes		Legs, +2
	76 F	2	8	10	Dead	Pain	Yes	Yes	Yes		Legs, –4

Intramedullary Tumors of the Spinal Cord (Continued)

Cerebrospinal Fluid			X-ray Diagnostic for Intra-spinal Tumor	Myelogram Diagnostic for Tumor, Spinal Cord	Location According to Vertebral Level	Syringomyelia: Cystic Surgical Lesion, With or Without Histologic Proof	Treatment		Comments
Protein, mg. per 100 cc.	Cells, no. per cu. mm.	Block of Fluid					X-ray	Surgical	
Dry			Yes	Yes	Lumbar 3–4		Yes	Total removal	
40	1		No		Lumbar 3–4			Total removal	
200	2		No		Lumbar 3–5			Total removal	Spina bifida occulta
			No		Lumbar 3–5		Yes	Total removal	Re-operation 3 yr. later
320	6		No		Lumbar 4–5			Total removal	
90	1		No	Yes	Lumbar 4–5			Total removal	
275	5		Yes		Lumbar 4–?			Biopsy, decompression	
			Yes		Lumbar 4 to sacral 2			?	
60	1		No		Lumbar 4 to sacral 4		Yes	Subtotal removal	
70			No	Yes	Lumbar 5 to sacral 1		Yes	Biopsy, decompression	
300	1		No	Yes	Lumbar 5 to sacral 1		Yes	Total removal	Spina bifida; Re-operation 2 yr. later
220	2		Yes		Lumbar 5 to sacral 4		Yes	Subtotal removal	Re-operation 8 yr. later; died, metastasis
Ependymomas, grade 3									
240	6				Thoracic 2–4			Subtotal removal, decompression	
7500	3		No	Yes	Thoracic 10 to lumbar 2		Yes	Subtotal removal	

Reported in Text as Case Number	Age, Years; Sex	Duration, Months			Living or Dead	Initial	Pain	Sensory Disturbance	Motor Disturbance	Bladder, Bowel Dysfunction	Reflexes, Grade
		Preoperative	Postoperative	Total							
	69 M	17	11	28	Alive, 1959	Bladder, bowel dysfunction	No	Yes	No	Yes	Legs, −4
	11 F	13	60	73	Alive, 1960	Pain	Yes	Yes	Yes		Legs, −4
	30 M	1	60	61	?	Pain	Yes	Yes	No		−

Recklinghausen's disease with intramedullary tumor: cases 34, 35, 3(

						Oligodendrogliomas					
32	45 F	15	−	−	Dead	Pain	Yes	Yes	Yes	Yes	Legs, −1
	40 M	48	30	78	Dead	Pain	Yes	Yes	Yes		Legs, +2
	36 M	9	348	357	Alive, 1960	Pain	Yes	Yes	Yes		Legs, −2
	52 M	7	24	31	Dead	Pain	Yes	Yes	Yes		Legs, +1
33	29 F	20	5	25	Dead	Pain	Yes	Yes	Yes	Yes	Legs, −4
	42 M	120	76	196	Dead	Pain	Yes	Yes	Yes		Legs, +2
	18 F	15	−	−	?	Pain	Yes	No	No		Legs, −3
	40 M	30	264	294	Alive, 1960	Pain	Yes	No	Yes		Legs, −2
						Mixed gliomas					
	20 F	2	2	4	Dead	Pain	Yes	Yes	Yes		Legs, +2
	40 F	180	228	408	Alive, 1960	Pain	Yes	No	Yes		Legs, −3
	18 F	3-1/2	228	331	Alive, 1960	Pain	Yes	Yes	No		Legs, −2

Intramedullary Tumors of the Spinal Cord (Continued)

Cerebrospinal Fluid			X-ray Diagnostic for Intra-spinal Tumor	Myelogram Diagnostic for Tumor, Spinal Cord	Location According to Vertebral Level	Syringomyelia: Cystic Surgical Lesion, With or Without Histo-logic Proof	Treatment		Comments
Protein, mg. per 100 cc.	Cells, no. per cu. mm.	Block of Fluid					X-ray	Surgical	
50	1		No	No	Thoracic 12 to lumbar 2			Total removal	Carcinoma, bladder
5000			No		Thoracic 12 to lumbar 3		Yes	Total removal	Scoliosis
200	1		No	Yes	Lumbar 2-3			Total removal	Re-operation 9 mo. later

nd 37 reported in full in Chapter IV, "Von Recklinghausen's Disease," p. 167.

					Oligodendrogliomas				
2400	2	Yes	Yes		Cervical 2-5			Subtotal removal	Surgical death
	23	Par-tial block	No		Cervical 3-7		Yes	Biopsy, decompression	
160	3	Par-tial block	No		Cervical 4-5			Total removal	
			Yes		Thoracic 4-5			Biopsy	
	6	Yes	No	Yes	Thoracic 5-11	With		Biopsy	Papilledema before death
280	1	Par-tial block			Thoracic 8-11		Yes	Subtotal removal	Papilledema, re-operation 6 yr. later
5000	1	Yes		Yes	Lumbar 1-3		Yes	Subtotal removal	
400	10		No		Lumbar 2-3		Yes	Total removal	

					Mixed gliomas				
7500		Yes	No		Cervical 5 to thoracic 3			Subtotal removal	Scoliosis; hemolytic anemia
			Yes		Thoracic 12 to sacral 1		Yes	Total removal	
			No	Yes	Sacral 2-4		Yes	Total removal	Re-operation twice, 1 and 12 yr. later

Reported in Text as Case Number	Age, Years; Sex	Duration, Months			Living or Dead	Symptoms					Reflexes, Grade
		Preoperative	Postoperative	Total		Initial	Pain	Sensory Disturbance	Motor Disturbance	Bladder, Bowel Dysfunction	
Subependymal glioma											
	48 M	72	18	90	Dead	Impotence	No	Yes	Yes		Legs, -3
Polar spongioblastoma											
18	46	7			Dead	Headache	Yes	Yes	No		–
Vascular tumors											
38	48 M	10	–	–	Dead	Pain	Yes	No	No		Legs, -4
39	30 M	120	–	–	Dead	Sensory disturbance	Yes	Yes	Yes		Arms, -2
40	30 F	60	–	–	Dead	Pain	Yes	Yes	Yes		Legs, +2
	13 F	3-1/2	68-1/2	72	Alive, 1960	Pain	Yes	No	No		–
	30 M	18	84	102	Dead	Pain	Yes	Yes	Yes		Legs, +1
	30 M	6	432	438	Dead	Pain	Yes	Yes	Yes		Legs, +2
	48 F	96	4	100	Dead	Motor disturbance	No	Yes	Yes		Legs, +2
	50 M	48	228	276	Dead	Pain	Yes	Yes	Yes		Legs, +2
41	32 M	48	–	–	Dead	Pain	Yes	Yes	Yes		Legs, +1
	51 M	4	100	104	Dead	Pain	Yes	No	?		Legs, +2
Sarcoma											
10	40 M	2	8	10	Alive, 1960	Pain	Yes	Yes	Yes		Legs, -1

Cerebrospinal Fluid			X-ray Diagnostic for Intra-spinal Tumor	Myelogram Diagnostic for Tumor, Spinal Cord	Location According to Vertebral Level	Syringomyelia: Cystic Surgical Lesion, With or Without Histologic Proof	Treatment		Comments
Protein, mg. per 100 cc.	Cells, no. per cu. mm.	Block of Fluid					X-ray	Surgical	
Subependymal glioma									
500	11		No	Yes	Thoracic 11 to lumbar 1	With	Yes	Biopsy	
Polar spongioblastoma									
850	11		No		Cervical 3 to thoracic 2	With			Papilledema
Vascular tumors									
4000	1		No		Cervical 3-4	With			Lindau's disease; papilledema
400	1	Yes			Cervical 3-6	With	Yes	Biopsy, decompression	
	6	Yes	No		Cervical 2-5 thoracic 1-2	With		Decompression	Lindau's disease
750	1	Yes	No	Yes	Cervical 4 to thoracic 1		Yes	Biopsy	
			No		Thoracic 2-3		Yes	Subtotal removal	
	9		No		Thoracic 4-6		Yes	Total removal	Stroke
60	1		Yes		Thoracic 6-7		Yes	Total removal	
400	8	Yes	No		Thoracic 6-8		Yes	Biopsy	Carcinoma, colon
			No		Thoracic 12	With			Lindau's disease
			No	Yes	Lumbar 4 to sacral 1			Total removal	Heart attack? Stroke?
Sarcoma									
6000	39		No	Yes	Lumbar 2-4		Yes	Total removal	Cordectomy 4 mo. later

Reported in Text as Case Number	Age, Years; Sex	Duration, Months			Living or Dead	Symptoms					Reflexes, Grade
		Preop- erative	Postop- erative	Total		Initial	Pain	Sensory Disturb- ance	Motor Disturb- ance	Bladder, Bowel Dys- function	
						Epidermoids, dermoids					
	35 M	120	96	216	Alive, 1960	Bladder, bowel dysfunction	No	Yes	Yes	Yes	Legs, −2
	40 M	120	?	?	Dead	Pain	Yes	Yes	Yes	Yes	Legs, −4
	61 M	120	–	–	Alive, 1960	Motor disturbance	No	Yes	Yes	Yes	Legs, −3
	32 F	204	240	444	Alive, 1960	Bladder, bowel dysfunction	Yes	Yes	No	Yes	Legs, −4
	21 F	4	216	220	Alive, 1960	Pain	Yes	Yes	No	Yes	Legs, −4
	30 M	24	156	180	Alive, 1959	Motor disturbance	Yes	Yes	Yes	No	Legs, −2
	45 M	96	48	144	Alive, 1960	Pain	Yes	Yes	Yes	Yes	Legs, −3
	44 F	180	204	384	Alive, 1959	Pain	Yes	Yes	No	Yes	Legs, +1
						Teratomas					
	20 M	3	108	111	Alive, 1960	Pain	Yes	No	Yes	No	Legs, +1
42	67 M	–	–	–	Dead						
						Lipomas					
	61 F	168	36	204	Alive, 1960	Pain	Yes	Yes	Yes		Legs, +1
	19 M	156	396	552	Alive, 1960	Pain	Yes	Yes	Yes		Arms, −2

Cerebrospinal Fluid			X-ray Diagnostic for Intra-spinal Tumor	Myelogram Diagnostic for Tumor, Spinal Cord	Location According to Vertebral Level	Syringomyelia: Cystic Surgical Lesion, With or Without Histo-logic Proof	Treatment		Comments
Protein, mg. per 100 cc.	Cells, no. per cu. mm.	Block of Fluid					X-ray	Surgical	
Epidermoids, dermoids									
55	2		No	Yes	Thoracic 11 to lumbar 2			Subtotal removal	Re-operation 8 yr. later; dermoid
440	8	Par-tial block		Yes	Thoracic 12 to lumbar 2			Subtotal removal	Dermoid
200	1		No	Yes	Thoracic 12 to lumbar 3			Total removal	Operation 6 yr. before; epidermoid
			Yes		Thoracic 12 to lumbar 3			Subtotal removal	Epidermoid
50	5		No	Yes	Lumbar 1-2			Subtotal removal	Dermoid
10	1		No	Yes	Lumbar 1-4			Subtotal removal	Re-operation 13 yr. later; spondylolis-thesis; dermoid
400	1	Yes	Yes	Yes	Lumbar 2-4			Biopsy, decompression	Epidermoid
20	1	Yes	?		Lumbar 3-5			Total removal	Epidermoid
Teratomas									
40	2	Yes	Yes	Yes	Thoracic 11 to lumbar 3			Total removal	
					Thoracic 12	With			Incidental finding
Lipomas									
65	1		No	Yes	Cervical 1-6			Subtotal removal, decompression	
	4	Par-tial block			Cervical 3-7		Yes	Subtotal removal	

235

Reported in Text as Case Number	Age, Years; Sex	Duration, Months			Living or Dead	Symptoms					
		Preop- erative	Postop- erative	Total		Initial	Pain	Sensory Disturb- ance	Motor Disturb- ance	Bladder, Bowel Dys- function	Reflexes, Grade
	22 M	45	180	225	Alive, 1958	Pain	Yes	No	Yes		Arms, -2
	8 M	48		?	?	Pain	Yes	No	Yes	Yes	Legs, -4
	45 M	48	72	120	Alive, 1960	?	?	Yes	Yes		Legs, + -
	56 M	372	60	462	Alive, 1960	Sensory disturbance	Yes	Yes	Yes		Legs, -3
Neurilemmoma											
	12 M	48	?	?	?	Pain	Yes	Yes	Yes		Arms, -4
Unclassified											
	20 F	48	3	51	Dead	Motor disturbance	Yes	Yes	Yes		Legs, -4

Cerebrospinal Fluid			X-ray Diagnostic for Intra-spinal Tumor	Myelogram Diagnostic for Tumor, Spinal Cord	Location According to Vertebral Level	Syringomyelia: Cystic Surgical Lesion, With or Without Histo-logic Proof	Treatment		Comments
Protein, mg. per 100 cc.	Cells, no. per cu. mm.	Block of Fluid					X-ray	Surgical	
1000	2	Partial block	No	Yes	Thoracic 2-5			Biopsy, decompression	
120	1		No	Yes	Thoracic 12 to lumbar 3			Subtotal removal, decompression	Spina bifida occulta
30	1		No	Yes	Lumbar 2-5			Subtotal removal	
40	1		Yes	?	Lumbar 3-4			Biopsy, decompression	Spina bifida occulta
Neurilemmoma									
			No		Cervical 4-7			Subtotal removal, decompression	
Unclassified									
			No		Thoracic 8 to lumbar 1			Biopsy, decompression	

BIBLIOGRAPHY

1. Adson, A. W.: Intraspinal Tumors; Surgical Consideration: Collective Review. Internat. Abstr. Chir. **67**:225–237 (Sept.) 1938.
2. Adson, A. W., and Ott, W. O.: Results of the Removal of Tumors of the Spinal Cord. Arch. Neurol. & Psychiat. **8**:520–537 (Nov.) 1922.
3. Alajouanine, T., and Theurel, R.: Syringomyélie, gliome et épendymome intra-médullaires. Rev. neurol. **73**:239–243 (May) 1941.
4. Allen, I.: Glioma of the Cervical Cord. Canad. M. A. J. **28**:417–420 (Apr.) 1933.
5. Anderson, F. M., and Carson, M. J.: Spinal Cord Tumors in Children: A Review of the Subject and Presentation of Twenty-one Cases. J. Pediat. **43**:190–207 (Aug.) 1953.
6. Austin, G. M.: The Significance and Nature of Pain in Tumors of the Spinal Cord. S. Forum. **10**:782–785, 1960.
7. Ayer, J. B.: Symptoms and Signs of Tumors Involving the Spinal Cord. New England J. Med. **203**:295–300 (Aug. 14) 1930.
8. Ayres, W. W.: Ependymoma of the Cauda Equina: A Report of the Clinico-pathologic Aspects and Follow-up Studies of 18 Cases. Mil. Med. **122**:10–35 (Jan.) 1958.
9. Bailey, P.: A Study of Tumors Arising From Ependymal Cells. Arch. Neurol. & Psychiat. **11**:1–27 (Jan.) 1924.
10. Bailey, P.: Quelques nouvelles observations de tumeurs épendymaires. Ann. anat. path. **2**:481–512 (Nov.) 1925.
11. Bailey, P.: Further Remarks Concerning Tumors of the Glioma Group. Bull. Johns Hopkins Hosp. **40**:354–389, 1927.
12. Bailey, P.: Cellular Types in Primary Tumors of the Brain. In Penfield, W.: Cytology and Cellular Pathology of the Nervous System. New York, Paul B. Hoeber, Inc., 1932, vol. 3, pp. 905–951.
13. Bailey, P.: A Review of Modern Conceptions of the Structure and Classification of Tumors Derived From the Medullary Epithelium. J. belge neurol. et psychiat. **38**:759–782, 1938.
14. Bailey, P., and Bucy, P. C.: Oligodendrogliomas of the Brain. J. Path. & Bact. **32**:735–751, 1929.
15. Bailey, P., and Bucy, P. C.: Tumors of the Spinal Canal. S. Clin. North America. **10**:233–257 (Apr.) 1930.
16. Bailey, P., and Cushing, H.: A Classification of the Tumors of the Glioma Group on a Histogenetic Basis With a Correlated Study of Prognosis. Philadelphia, J. B. Lippincott Co., 1926.

239

17. Bailey, P., and Hiller, G.: The Interstitial Tissues of the Central Nervous System: A Review. J. Nerv. & Ment. Dis. **59**:337–361 (Apr.) 1924.
18. Bergstrand, H.: Weiteres über sogenannte Kleinhirnastrocytome. Virchows Arch. f. path. Anat. **299**:725–739, 1937.
19. Berkwitz, N. J.: Extensive Longitudinal Cavitation of the Spinal Cord Associated With a Circumscribed Intramedullary Tumor. Arch. Neurol. & Psychiat. **32**: 569–576 (Sept.) 1934.
20. Besold, G.: Ueber zwei Fälle von Gehirntumor (Hämangiosarkom oder sogenanntes Peritheliom in der Gegend des dritten Ventrikels) bei zwei Geschwistern. Deutsche Ztschr. Nervenh. **8**:49–74, 1896.
21. Bielschowsky, M., and Unger, E.: Syringomyelie mit Teratom-und extramedullärer Blastombildung. J. f. Psychol. u. Neurol. **25**:173–218, 1920.
22. Bors, E.: Sacral Neurotomy or Low Subarachnoid Alcohol Block in Autonomic Hyperreflexia, in discussion on Kurnick, N. B.: Drug Therapy of Autonomic Hyperreflexia in Patients With Spinal Cord Lesions, read at the Third Annual Paraplegia Conference, Veterans Administration Hospital, West Roxbury, Mass. Oct. 12–14, 1954.
23. Bostroem, E.: Ueber die pialen Epidermoide, Dermoide und Lipome und duralen Dermoide. Zentralbl. allg. Path. **8**:1–98 (Jan.) 1897.
24. Boykin, F. C., Cowen, D., Iannucci, C. A. J., and Wolf, A.: Subependymal Glomerate Astrocytomas. J. Neuropath. & Exper. Neurol. **13**:30–49 (Jan.) 1954.
25. Boyle, J. B., Jr.: A Clinical-Pathological Study of Von Recklinghausen's Disease. Thesis, Graduate School, University of Minnesota, 1958.
26. Bradford, F. K.: Intramedullary Dermoid Cyst. Ann. Surg. **107**:107–115 (Jan.) 1938.
27. Bradford, F. K.: Intraspinal Tumors. Dis. Nerv. System. **15**:55–60 (Feb.) 1954.
28. Bremer, F. W.: Die pathologisch-anatomische Begründung des Status dysraphicus. Deutsche Ztschr. Nervenh. **99**:104–123, 1927.
29. Bremer, F. W.: Syringomyelie. Fortschr. d. Neurol., Psychiat. **1**:429–437, 1929.
30. Brizzi, R.: Intraspinal Dermoids: Report of Three Cases. Acta neurochir. **4**:164–170, 1955.
31. Broager, B.: Spinal Neurinoma. Acta psychiat. et neurol. Suppl. 85, 1953.
32. Browder, J.: Tumors of the Spinal Cord. Am. J. Surg. **24**:1–10 (Apr.) 1934.
33. Brown, R. W.: The Central Canal of the Spinal Cord. Thesis, Graduate School, University of Minnesota, 1939.
34. Buchanan, D.: Tumors of the Spinal Cord in Infancy. (Abstr.) Arch. Neurol. & Psychiat. **63**:835 (May) 1950.
35. Bucy, P. C., and Buchanan, D. N.: Teratoma of the Spinal Cord. Surg., Gynec. & Obst. **60**:1137–1144 (June) 1935.
36. Bucy, P. C., and Gustafson, W. A.: Structure, Nature and Classification of the Cerebellar Astrocytomas. Am. J. Cancer. **35**:327–353 (Mar.) 1939.
37. Bunts, A. T.: Spinal Cord Tumors: An Analytical Review of 36 Cases. S. Clin. North America. **15**:1047–1062 (Aug.) 1935.
38. Bunts, A. T.: The Mimicry of Tumors of the Spinal Cord. Am. Surgeon. **26**:630–633 (Sept.) 1960.
39. Bunschor, O.: Über den sogenannten Syringomyeliekomplex unter besonderer Berücksichtigung der Hydromyelie. Confinia neurol. **19**:21–40, 1959.
40. Cairns, H., and Riddoch, G.: Observations on the Treatment of Ependymal Gliomas of the Spinal Cord. Brain. **54**:117–146 (June) 1931.
41. Cajal, S.: Nouvelles observations sur l'évolution des neuroblastes, avec quelques remarques sur l'hypothèse neurogénétique de Hensen-Held. Anat. Anz. **32**:1–25 (Jan. 7); 65–87 (Jan. 21) 1908.
42. Camp, J. D.: The Roentgenologic Localization of Tumors Affecting the Spinal Cord. Am. J. Roentgenol. **40**:540–544 (Oct.) 1958.
43. Canti, R. G., Bland, J. O. W., and Russell, D. S.: Tissue Culture of Gliomata. A. Res. Nerv. & Ment. Dis., Proc. **16**:1–23, 1937.
44. Caram, P. C., Scarcella, G., and Carton, C. A.: Intradural Lipomas of the Spinal Cord. J. Neurosurg. **14**:28–42, 1957.
45. Chason, J. L.: Subependymal Mixed Gliomas. J. Neuropath. & Exper. Neurol. **15**: 461–470 (Oct.) 1956.

46. Chiasson, S. W., and Corkran, R. G.: Syringomyelia. McGill M. J. 14:65–79 (Feb.) 1945.
47. Collins, J., and Marks, H. E.: The Early Diagnosis of Spinal Cord Tumors. Am. J. M. Sc. 149:103–112 (Jan.) 1915.
48. Cooper, I. S., Craig, W. McK., and Kernohan, J. W.: Tumors of the Spinal Cord: Primary Extramedullary Gliomas. Collect. Papers Mayo Clin. 42:493–495, 1950.
49. Cooper, I. S., and Hoen, T. I.: Gynecomastia in Paraplegic Males: Report of Seven Cases. J. Clin. Endocrinol. 9:457–461 (May) 1949.
50. Cooper, I. S., and Hoen, T. I.: Intrathecal Alcohol in the Treatment of Spastic Paraplegia. J. Neurosurg. 6:187–190 (May) 1949.
51. Cooper, I. S., Kernohan, J. W., and Craig, W. McK.: Tumors of the Medulla Oblongata. Arch. Neurol. & Psychiat. 67:269–282, 1952.
52. Cooper, I. S., MacCarty, C. S., Rynearson, E. H., and Bennett, W. A.: Metabolic Consequences of Spinal Cordectomy. Proc. Staff Meet., Mayo Clin. 24:620–627 (Dec. 7) 1949.
53. Cooper, I. S., Rynearson, E. H., MacCarty, C. S., and Power, M. H.: Metabolic Consequences of Spinal Cord Injury. J. Clin. Endocrinol. 10:858–870 (Aug.) 1950.
54. Cornil, L., and Mosinger, M.: Sur les processus prolifératifs de l'épendyme médullaire (Rapports avec les tumeurs intramédullaires et la syringomyélie). Rev. Neurol. 1:749–754 (May) 1933.
55. Courville, C.: Quoted by Poser, C. M.[217]
56. Cox, L. B.: The Cytology of the Glioma Group; With Special Reference to the Inclusion of Cells Derived From the Invaded Tissue. Am. J. Path. 9:839–898 (Nov.) 1933.
57. Cox, L. B.: A Case of Syringomyelia Associated With an Intra-medullary Tumour, With Remarks on the Relation of the Gliosis to Tumours of Ependymal Origin. J. Path. & Bact. 44:661–678 (May) 1937.
58. Craig, W. McK.: Spinal Cord Compression: Tumors and Allied Non-traumatic Conditions. Am. J. Surg. 12:303–313 (May) 1931.
59. Craig, W. McK.: The Pain of Tumors of the Spinal Cord. West. J. Surg. 40:56–63 (Feb.) 1932
60. Craig, W. McK.: Experimental Production of the Syndrome of Spinal Cord Tumors. S. Clin. North America. 13:915–926 (Aug.) 1933.
61. Craig, W. McK., and Shelden, C. H.: Tumors of the Cervical Portion of the Spinal Cord. Arch. Neurol. & Psychiat. 44:1–16 (July) 1940.
62. Craig, W. M., Svien, H. J., and Mabon, R. F.: Surgical Application. Proc. Staff Meet., Mayo Clin. 24:76–77 (Feb.) 1949.
63. Craig, W. McK., and Horras, G.: The Occurrence of Hemangioblastomas (Two Cerebellar and One Spinal) in Three Members of a Family. J. Neurosurg. 6:518–529 (Dec.) 1949.
64. Craig, W. McK., Wagener, H. P., and Kernohan, J. W.: Lindau von Hippel Disease. Arch. Neurol. & Psychiat. 46:36–54, 1941.
65. Crosby, R. M. N., Wagner, J. A., and Nichols, P.: Intradural Lipoma of the Spinal Cord. J. Neurosurg. 10:81–86, 1953.
66. Cushing, H., and Bailey, P.: Tumors Arising From the Blood-Vessels of the Brain; Angiomatous Malformations and Hemangioblastomas. Springfield, Ill., Charles C Thomas, Publisher, 1928.
67. De Busscher, J., Scherer, H. J., and Thomas, F.: Recklinghausen's Neurofibromatosis Combined With True Syringomyelia. J. belge neurol. et psychiat. 38:788–802, 1938.
68. Denk, W.: Diagnose und Therapie der Rückenmarkstumoren. Cong. Soc. internat. de chir. 2:445–478, 1932.
69. Dodge, H. W., Keith, H. M., and Campagna, M. J.: Intraspinal Tumors in Infants and Childhood. J. Internat. Coll. Surgeons. 26:199–215, 1956.
70. Dunn, A. W., and Aponte, G. E.: Ependymoma of the Conus Medullaris. U. S. Armed Forces M. J. 11:341–346 (Mar.) 1960.
71. Earnest, F., III, Kernohan, J. W., and Craig, W. McK.: Oligodendrogliomas: A Review of Two Hundred Cases. Arch. Neurol. & Psychiat. 63:964–976 (June) 1950.

72. Eaton, L. McK.: Pain Caused by Disease Involving the Sensory Nerve Roots (Root Pain). J.A.M.A. 117:1435–1439 (Oct. 25) 1941.
73. Ebbers, H.: Über das gleichzeitige Vorkommen von Syringomyelie mit Recklinghausenscher Krankheit und Hirntumor. Arch. Psychiat. 113:605–618 (Aug.) 1941.
74. Ehni, G.: Intraspinal and Intracranial Lipomas: Report of Cases, Review of the Literature, and Clinical and Pathological Study of Intraspinal Lipomas With Report of Cases and Discussion of Intracranial Lipomas. Thesis, Graduate School, University of Minnesota, 1943.
75. Ehni, G., and Love, J. G.: Intraspinal Lipomas: Report of Cases; Review of the Literature, and Clinical and Pathologic Study. Arch. Neurol. & Psychiat. 53:1–28 (Jan.) 1945.
76. Eiselsberg, A.: Intramedulläre Rückenmarkstumoren. Mitt. a.d. Grenzgeb. d. Med. u. Chir. 42:613–622, 1931.
77. Eiselsberg, A. F., and Ranzi, E.: Ueber die chirurgische Behandlung der Hirn- und Rückenmarkstumoren. Arch. f. klin. chir. 102:309–468 (Sept.) 1913.
78. Elsberg, C. A.: Tumors of the Spinal Cord: Problems in Their Diagnosis and Localization; Procedures for Their Exposure and Removal. Arch. Neurol. & Psychiat. 22:949–965, 1929.
79. Elsberg, C. A.: The Diagnosis and Surgical Treatment of Tumors of the Spinal Cord. Cong. Soc. internat. de chir. 2:385–444, 1932.
80. Elsberg, C. A.: Surgical Diseases of the Spinal Cord, Membranes and Nerve Roots: Symptoms, Diagnosis and Treatment. New York, Paul B. Hoeber, Inc., 1941.
81. Elsberg, C. A., and Dyke, C. G.: The Diagnosis and Localization of Tumors of the Spinal Cord by Means of Measurements Made on the X-ray Films of the Vertebrae, and the Correlation of Clinical and X-ray Findings. Bull. Neurol. Inst. New York. 3:359–394 (Mar.) 1934.
82. Elsberg, C. A., and Stookey, B.: The Mechanical Effects of Tumors of the Spinal Cord: Their Influence on Symptomatology and Diagnosis. Arch. Neurol. & Psychiat. 8:502–514 (Nov.) 1922.
83. Elvidge, A. R., and Martinez-Coll, A.: Long-term Follow-up of 106 Cases of Astrocytoma, 1928–1939. J. Neurosurg. 13:318–331 (July) 1956.
84. Elvidge, A., Penfield, W., and Cone, W.: The Gliomas of the Central Nervous System: A Study of Two Hundred and Ten Verified Cases. A Res. Nerv. & Ment. Dis., Proc. 16:107–181, 1937.
85. Eneström, S., and Gröntoft, O.: Oligodendroglioma of the Spinal Cord: Report of One Case. Acta path. et microbiol. scandinav. 40:396–400, 1957.
86. Ernst, P.: Quoted by Sperling, S. J., and Alpers, B. J.[268]
87. Farnarier, G., Roger, J., and Vigouroux, R.: Localisation médullaire d'un médulloblastome avec syndrome d' hypertension intra-cranienne. Rev. d'oto-neuro-opht. 29:490–494 (July) 1957.
88. Feller, A., and Sternberg, H.: Zur Kenntnis der Fehlbildungen der Wirbelsäule. I. Die Wirbelkörperspalte und ihre formale Genese. Virchows Arch. f. path. Anat. 272:613–640 (June) 1929.
89. Fincher, E. F.: Spontaneous Subarachnoid Hemorrhage in Intradural Tumors of the Lumbar Sac. J. Neurosurg. 8:576–584 (Nov.) 1951.
90. Fisher, D. A.: Embryonal Rest Tumor of the Central Nervous System: Report of an Unusual Case With a Communicating Congenital Dermal Sinus and Recurrent Meningitis. A.M.A. J. Dis. Child. 99:90–97 (Jan.) 1960.
91. Flock, H.: Über die Häufigkeit der Gliome. Frankfurt. Ztschr. f. Path. 50:289–303, 1936–1937.
92. Foerster, A.: Ein Ganglioneurom des Rückenmarks. Virchows Arch. f. path. Anat. 253:116–124, 1924.
93. Foerster, O., and Bailey, P.: A Contribution to the Study of Gliomas of the Spinal Cord With Special Reference to Their Operability. In Jubilee Volume for Dawindenkow. Leningrad State Institute for the Publication of Biological and Medical Literature, 1936, pp. 9–67.
94. Foerster, O., and Gagel, O.: Klinik und Pathohistologie der intramedullären Rückenmarkstumoren. Deutsche Ztschr. f. Nervenh. 136:239–240 (Mar.) 1935.

95. Ford, F. R.: Diseases of the Nervous System in Infancy, Childhood and Adolescence. Ed. 2, Springfield, Ill., Charles C Thomas, Publisher, 1960.

96. Frazier, C. H., and Alpers, B. J.: The Effect of Irradiation on the Gliomas. In Tumors of the Nervous System. A. Res. Nerv. & Ment. Dis., Proc. 16:68–106, 1937.

97. Frazier, C. H., and Spiller, W. G.: An Analysis of Fourteen Consecutive Cases of Spinal Cord Tumor. Arch. Neurol. & Psychiat. 8:455–501 (Nov.) 1922.

98. French, L. A., and Peyton, W. T.: Mixed Tumors of the Spinal Canal. Arch. Neurol. & Psychiat. 47:737–751 (May) 1942.

99. Furtado, D., and Marques, V.: Spinal Teratoma. J. Neuropath. & Exper. Neurol. 10:384–393 (Oct.) 1951.

100. Gagel, O.: Über Hirngeschwülste. Ztschr. f. d. ges. Neurol. u. Psychiat. 161:69–113, 1938.

101. Gagnon, J., and Courtois, A.: Syringomyélie de l'enfant associée à une tumeur intra-médullaire: Contribution à l'hypothèse de Kirch. Acta neurol. et psychiat. belg. 60:1037–1053, 1960.

102. Gallagher, J. P.: Malignant Neoplasms of the Central Nervous System: Tumors of the Spinal Cord. M. Ann. District of Columbia. 2:45–48 (June) 1950.

103. Gardner, W. J., Spitler, D. K., and Whitten, C.: Increased Intracranial Pressure Caused by Increased Protein Content in the Cerebrospinal Fluid: An Explanation of Papilledema in Certain Cases of Small Intracranial and Intraspinal Tumors and in the Guillain-Barré Syndrome. New England J. Med. 250:932–936 (June) 1954.

104. Globus, J. H., and Doshay, L. J.: Venous Dilatations and Other Intraspinal Vessel Alterations, Including True Angiomata, With Signs and Symptoms of Cord Compression: A Report of Four Cases With a Review of the Literature. Surg., Gynec. & Obst. 48:345–366 (Mar.) 1929.

105. Globus, J. H., and Strauss, I.: Spongioblastoma Multiforme: A Primary Malignant Form of Brain Neoplasm: Its Clinical and Anatomic Features. Arch. Neurol. & Psychiat. 14:139–191 (Aug.) 1925.

106. Gowers, W. R., and Horsley, V. A.: A Case of Tumour of the Spinal Cord; Removal: Recovery. Tr. Med. Chir. Soc. Edinburgh. 71:379–430, 1888.

107. Grant, F. C.: Successful Removal of a Large Intramedullary Tumor of the Spinal Cord. Arch. Neurol. & Psychiat. 52:157–158 (Aug.) 1944.

108. Grant, F. C., and Austin, G. M.: The Diagnosis, Treatment, and Prognosis of Tumors Affecting the Spinal Cord in Children. J. Neurosurg. 13:535–545 (Nov.) 1956.

109. Grcevic, N., and Yates, P. O.: Rosenthal Fibres in Tumours of the Central Nervous System. J. Path. & Bact. 73:467–472 (Apr.) 1957.

110. Greenfield, J. G., Blackwood, W., McMenemey, W. H., Meyer, A., and Norman, R. M.; Neuropathology. London, Edward Arnold, Ltd., 1958.

111. Greenwood, J., Jr.: Total Removal of Intramedullary Tumors. J. Neurosurg. 11:616–621 (Nov.) 1954.

112. Grossman, M.: Syringomyelia: Clinical Report of Ten Cases, Illustrating Spinal, Bulbar, and Congenital Types of the Disease, With Anatomic Confirmation in Three Instances. J. Mt. Sinai Hosp. 9:526–535 (Nov.–Dec.) 1942.

113. Haft, H., Ransohoff, J., and Carter, S.: Spinal Cord Tumors in Children. Pediatrics. 23:1152–1159 (June) 1959.

114. Hallopeau: Quoted by Simon, T.[265]

115. Hamby, W. B.: Tumors in the Spinal Canal in Childhood. J. Nerv. & Ment. Dis. 81:24–42 (Jan.) 1935.

116. Hamby, W. B.: Tumors in the Spinal Canal in Childhood: Analysis of the Literature of a Subsequent Decade (1933–1942); Report of a Case of Meningitis Due to an Intramedullary Epidermoid Communicating With a Dermal Sinus. J. Neuropath. & Exper. Neurol. 3:397–412 (Oct.) 1944.

117. Hamilton, P. K.: Neuroblastoma of the Spinal Cord. Am. J. Clin. Path. 21:846–851 (Sept.) 1951.

118. Harmeier, J. W.: The Normal Histology of the Intradural Filum Terminale. Arch. Neurol. & Psychiat. 29:308–316 (Feb.) 1933.

119. Harriman, D. G. F.: An Intraspinal Enterogenous Cyst. J. Path. & Bact. 75:413–419 (Apr.) 1958.

120. Henneberg, R., and Koch, M.: Zur Pathogenese der Syringomyelie und über Häma-
     tomyelie bei Syringomyelie. Monatsschr. Psychiat. u. Neurol. **54**:117–140, 1923.
121. Henschen, F.: Tumoren des Zentralnervensystems und seiner Hüllen. In Henke, F.,
     and Lubarsch, O.: Handbuch der Speziellen Pathologischen Anatomie und
     Histologie. vol. 13, 1955, pp. 413–1040.
122. Hepburn, A. L.: Recurrent Ependymomas: A Clinical Pathological Study. Thesis,
     Graduate School, University of Minnesota, 1956.
123. Hoff, H., and Weingarten, K.: Ueber spinale Tumoren im Kindesalter. Wien. klin.
     Wchnschr. **64**:220–222 (Mar. 21) 1952.
124. Holmdahl, D. E.: Die Zweifache Bildungsweise des Zentralen Nervensystems bei
     den Wirbeltieren. Arch. f. Entwicklungsmech. d. Organ. **129**:206–254 (June)
     1933.
125. Horrax, G., and Henderson, D. G.: Encapsulated Intramedullary Tumor Involving
     the Whole Spinal Cord From Medulla to Conus: Complete Enucleation With
     Recovery. Surg., Gynec. & Obst. **68**:814–819 (Apr.) 1939.
126. Hosci, K.: Intradural Teratoid Tumors of the Spinal Cord: Report of a Case. Arch.
     Path. **11**:875–883 (June) 1931.
127. Hurteau, E. F., Baird, W. C., and Sinclair, E.: Arachnoiditis Following the Use of
     Iodized Oil. J. Bone & Joint Surg. **36–A**:393–400 (Apr.) 1954.
128. Ingebrigtsen, R., and Leegaard, T.: Final Results in a Series of Operated Intra-
     spinal Tumors. Acta chir. scandinav. **82**:271–281, 1939.
129. Ingraham, F. D.: Intraspinal Tumors in Infancy and Childhood. Am. J. Surg.
     39:342–376 (Feb.) 1938.
130. Ingraham, F. D., and Bailey, O. T.: Cystic Teratomas and Teratoid Tumors of the
     Central Nervous System in Infancy and Children. J. Neurosurg. **3**:511–532 (Nov.)
     1946.
131. Ingraham, F. D., and Matson, D. D.: Neurosurgery of Infancy and Childhood.
     Springfield, Ill., Charles C. Thomas, Publisher, 1954.
132. Jackson, R. B.: Intramedullary Hemangioma of the Spinal Cord. California Med.
     87:41–44 (July) 1957.
133. Jirasek, A.: Diagnosis and Treatment of Intraspinal Tumors. Cong. Soc. internat. de
     chir. **2**:667–711, 1932.
134. Joffroy, A., and Achard: De la myélite cavitaire. Arch. de physiol. norm. et path.
     Série III. **10**:435–472, 1887.
135. Joffroy, A., and Achard, Ch.: Syringomyélie non gliomateuse associée à la maladie
     de Basedow. Arch. de méd. expér. et d'anat. path. **3**:91–108, 1891.
136. Johnson, D. F.: Intramedullary Lipoma of the Spinal Cord: Review of the Litera-
     ture and Report of Case. Bull. Los Angeles Neurol. Soc. **15**:37–42 (Mar.) 1950.
137. Jones, O. W., and Naffziger, H. C.: Tumors on the Spinal Cord: Their Diagnosis.
     California & West. Med. **45**:17–19 (July) 1936.
138. Jonesco-Sisesti, N.: Tumeurs médullaires associées à un processus syringomiélique.
     Paris, Masson & Cie, 1929.
139. Karavitis, A. L.: Ependymomas and Oligodendrogliomas of the Thoracic Portion
     of the Spinal Cord. Thesis, Graduate School, University of Minnesota, 1954.
140. Kernohan, J. W.: The Ventriculus Terminalis: Its Growth and Development. J.
     Comp. Neurol. **38**:107–125 (Dec.) 1924.
141. Kernohan, J. W.: Primary Tumors of the Spinal Cord and Intradural Filum Termi-
     nale. In Penfield, W.: Cytology and Cellular Pathology of the Nervous System.
     New York, Paul B. Hoeber, Inc., 1932, pp. 993–1025.
142. Kernohan, J. W.: Tumors of the Central Nervous System. Proc. Staff Meet., Mayo
     Clin. **13**:827–832 (Dec. 28) 1938.
143. Kernohan, J. W.: Tumors of the Spinal Cord. Arch. Path. **32**:843–882 (Nov.) 1941.
144. Kernohan, J. W., and Fletcher-Kernohan, E. M.: Ependymomas: A Study of 109
     Cases. A. Res. Nerv. & Ment. Dis., Proc. **16**:182–209, 1937.
145. Kernohan, J. W., Mabon, R. F., Svien, H. J., and Adson, A. W.: A Simplified Classi-
     fication of the Gliomas. Proc. Staff Meet., Mayo Clin. **24**:71–75 (Feb. 2) 1949.
146. Kernohan, J. W., and Parker, H. L.: A Case of Recklinghausen's Disease With Ob-
     servations on the Associated Formation of Tumors. J. Nerv. & Ment. Dis.
     76:313–330 (Oct.) 1932.
147. Kernohan, J. W., and Sayre, G. P.: Tumors of the Central Nervous System. In Atlas

of Tumor Pathology, National Research Council. Armed Forces Institute of Pathology, Washington, D.C., 1952.

148. Kernohan, J. W., and Sayre, G. P.: Tumours of the Central and Peripheral Nervous Systems. In Raven, R. W.: Cancer. London, Butterworth & Co., vol. 2, 1958, pp. 525–551.

149. Kernohan, J. W., and Uihlein, A.: Sarcomas of the Brain. Springfield, Ill., Charles C Thomas, Publisher, 1962.

150. Kernohan, J. W., Woltman, H. W., and Adson, A. W.: Intramedullary Tumors of the Spinal Cord: A Review of Fifty-one Cases, With an Attempt at Histologic Classification, Arch. Neurol. & Psychiat. 25:679–699 (Apr.) 1931.

151. Kernohan, J. W., Woltman, H. W., and Adson, A. W.: Gliomas Arising From the Region of the Cauda Equina. Arch. Neurol. & Psychiat. 29:287–305 (Feb.) 1933.

152. King, A. B.: Intramedullary Epidermoid Tumor of the Spinal Cord. J. Neurosurg. 14:353–357 (May) 1957.

153. Kinney, T. D., and Fitzgerald, P. J.: Lindau-Von Hippel Disease With Hemangioblastoma of the Spinal Cord and Syringomyelia. Arch. Path. 43:439–455 (May) 1947.

154. Kirch, E.: Über die Pathogenetischen Beziehungen zwischen Rückenmarksgeschwülsten und Syringomyelie. Ztschr. f. d. ges. Neurol. u. Psychiat. 117:231–287, 1928.

155. Kirgis, H. D., and Echols, D. H.: Syringo-encephalomyelia: Discussion of Related Syndromes and Pathologic Processes, With Report of a Case. J. Neurosurg. 6:368–375 (Sept.) 1949.

156. Knight, G., Griffiths, T., and Williams, I.: Gastrocystoma of the Spinal Cord. Brit. J. Surg. 42:635–638 (May) 1954–55.

157. Krabbe, K. H.: Les tumeurs intraspinales de l'enfance. Acta psychiat. et neurol. Suppl. 46, 1947, pp. 175–186.

158. Krayenbühl, H., and Lüthy, F.: Das spinale Neurinom und sympathische Ganglioneurom im Kindesalter. Schweiz. Ztschr. f. Path. u. Bakter. 10:51–65, 1947.

159. Kuntz, A.: A Text-book of Neuro-anatomy. Philadelphia, Lea & Febiger, 1950.

160. Kurland, L. T.: The Frequency of Intracranial and Intraspinal Neoplasms in the Resident Population of Rochester, Minnesota. J. Neurosurg. 15:627–641 (Nov.) 1958.

161. Kwan, S. T., and Alpers, B. J.: The Oligodendrogliomas: A Clinicopathologic Study. Arch. Neurol. & Psychiat. 26:279–321 (Aug.) 1931.

162. Landau, M.: Über Rückbildungsvorgänge in Gliomen. Frankfurt. Ztschr. Path. 7:351–372, 1911.

163. de Lange, C.: Fieber von 6½ jähriger Dauer bei einem Kinde mit angeborenen Missbildungen des Gehirns und Rückenmarks und angeborenem Tumor medullae. Acta Paed. 14:503–543, 1932–33.

164. Langhans, T.: Ueber Höhlenbildung im Rückenmark als Folge von Blutstauung. Virchows Arch. path. Anat. 85:1–25 (July) 1881.

165. Léchelle, P., Petit-Dutaillis, L., and Perset: Tumeurs multiples de la moelle cervicale de nature histologique différente: Évolution simultanée d'une localisation intracrânienne. Bull. et mém. Soc. med. d. hôp. de Paris. 1:343–348 (Mar. 9–23) 1956.

166. Lehoczky, T. de: Ependymoblastome spinal accompagné de syringomyélie. Acta neurol. et psychiat. belg. 49:1–12 (Jan.) 1949.

167. Lemmen, L. J., and Wilson, C. M.: Intramedullary Malignant Teratoma of the Spinal Cord, Arch. Neurol. & Psychiat. 66:61–68 (July) 1951.

168. Levaditi, C., Lépine, P., and Schoen, R.: Méchanisme pathogénique des formations cavitaires du névraxe: Porencéphalie et syringomyélie. Ann. Inst. Pasteur. 43:1465–1511 (Nov.) 1929.

169. Levaditi, C., Lépine, P., and Schoen, R.: Contribution expérimentale à l'étude étiologique de la syringomyélie. Bull. Acad. de méd., Paris. 101:669–680 (June) 1929.

170. Levy, L. F., and Elvidge, A. R.: Astrocytoma of the Brain and Spinal Cord. J. Neurosurg. 13:413–443 (Sept.) 1956.

171. Leyden, E.: Ueber Hydromyelie und Syringomyelie. Virchows Arch. path. Anat. 68:1–26 (Oct.) 1876.

172. Liber, A. F.: The Nature of Rosenthal Fibers. J. Nerv. & Ment. Dis. 85:286–304 (Mar.) 1937.

173. Liber, A. F., and Lisa, J. R.: Rosenthal Fibers in Non-neoplastic Syringomyelia: A Note on the Pathogenesis of Syringomyelia. J. Nerv. & Ment. Dis. 86:549–558 (Nov.) 1937.

174. Lichtenstein, B. W.: Multiple Primary Tumors of the Spinal Cord. Arch. Neurol. & Psychiat. 46:59–71 (July) 1941.

175. Lichtenstein, B. W., and Zeitlin, H.: Ganglioglioneuroma of Spinal Cord Associated With Pseudosyringomyelia: Histologic Study. Arch. Neurol. & Psychiat. 37:1356–1370 (June) 1937.

176. Lindau, A.: Studien über Kleinhirncysten: Bau, Pathogenese und Beziehungen zur Angiomatosis Retinae. Acta path. et microbiol. scandinav. Suppl. 1, 1926, 128 pp.

177. List, C. F.: Intraspinal Epidermoids, Dermoids, and Dermal Sinuses. Surg., Gynec. & Obst. 73:525–538 (Oct.) 1941.

178. Locoge, M.: Considérations sur la pathogénie des épidermodermoides et tératomes du système nerveux. Acta neurol. et psychiat. belg. 58:753–757, 1958.

179. Locoge, M., Brihaye, J., and Hasaerts, R.: Dysembryomes hétérotopiques de cône médullaire (avec révue de la littérature). Acta neurol. et psychiat. belg. 58:597–633, 1958.

180. Lombardi, G., and Migliavacoa, F.: Angiomas of the Spinal Cord. Brit. J. Radiol. 32:810–814 (Dec.) 1959.

181. Love, J. G., and Kernohan, J. W.: Dermoid and Epidermoid Tumors (Cholesteatomas) of Central Nervous System. J. A. M. A. 107:1876–1883 (Dec. 5) 1936.

182. Love, J. G., Wagener, H. P., and Woltman, H. W.: Tumors of the Spinal Cord Associated With Choking of the Optic Disks. Arch. Neurol. & Pyschiat. 66:171–177 (Aug.) 1951.

183. Lüthy, F., and Irsigler, F. J.: Beitrag zur Klinik und Histologie der Ependymome der Cauda Equina. Acta neurochir. 2:354–368 (July) 1952.

184. Mabon, R. F., Svien, H. J., Adson, A. W., and Kernohan, J. W.: Astrocytomas of the Cerebellum. Arch. Neurol. & Psychiat. 64:74–88 (July) 1950.

185. Mabon, R. F., Svien, H. J., Kernohan, J. W., and Craig, W. M.: Ependymomas. Proc. Staff Meet., Mayo Clin. 24:65–71 (Feb. 2) 1949.

186. MacCarty, C. S.: The Treatment of Spastic Paraplegia by Selective Spinal Cordectomy. J. Neurosurg. 11:539–545 (Nov.) 1954.

187. MacCarty, C. S., and Kiefer, E. J.: Thoracic, Lumbar and Sacral Spinal Cordectomy: Preliminary Report. Proc. Staff Meet., Mayo Clin. 24:108–115 (Feb. 16) 1949.

188. MacCarty, C. S., Leavens, M. E., Love, J. G., and Kernohan, J. W.: Dermoid and Epidermoid Tumors in the Central Nervous System of Adults. Surg., Gynec. & Obst. 108:191–198 (Feb.) 1959.

189. Mackay, R. P., and Favill, J.: Syringomyelia and Intramedullary Tumor of the Spinal Cord. Arch. Neurol. & Psychiat. 33:1255–1278 (June) 1935.

190. Mahoney, W.: Die Epidermoide des Zentralnervensystems. Ztschr. f. d. ges. Neurol. u. Psychiat. 155:416–471, 1936.

191. Mallory, F. B.: Three Gliomata of Ependymal Origin: Two in the Fourth Ventricle, One Subcutaneous Over the Coccyx. J. Med. Res. 8:1–10 (June) 1902.

192. McDonald, C. C.: Subependymal Glioma. Thesis, Graduate School, University of Minnesota, 1957.

193. Meirowsky, A. M., Scheibert, C. D., and Hinchey, T. R.: Studies on the Sacral Reflex Arc in Paraplegia. I. Response of the Bladder to Surgical Elimination of Sacral Nerve Impulses by Rhizotomy. J. Neurosurg. 7:33–43 (Jan.) 1950.

194. Mendelsohn, R. A., and Mora, F.: Spontaneous Subarachnoid Hemorrhage Caused by Ependymoma of Filum Terminale. J. Neurosurg. 15:460–463 (July) 1958.

195. Miura, K.: Ueber Gliom des Rückenmarks und Syringomyelie (Zugleick ein Beitrag zur aufsteigenden Degeneration der Schleife). Beitr. path. Anat. 11:91–124, 1892.

196. Moersch, F. P., Craig, W. McK., and Christoferson, L. A.: Spinal Cord Tumors With Minimal Neurologic Findings. Collect. Papers Mayo Clin. 42:496, 1950.

197. Mosberg, W. H.: Spinal Tumors Diagnosed During the First Year of Life With Report of a Case. J. Neurosurg. 8:220–224 (Mar.) 1951.

198. Munro, D.: Anterior-Rootlet Rhizotomy: A Method of Controlling Spasm With Retention of Voluntary Motion. New England J. Med. 246:161–166 (Jan. 31) 1952.

199. Muthmann, A., and Sauerbeck, E.: Ueber eine Gliageschwulst des IV Ventrikels (Neuroepithelioma gliomatosum columnocellulare veli medullaris posterioris) nebst allgemeinen Bemerkungen uber die Gliome uberhaupt. Beitr. path. Anat. 34:445–488, 1903.

200. Naciarone, A.: Quoted by Sperling, S. J., and Alpers, B. J.[268]

201. Netsky, M. G.: Syringomyelia: A Clinocopathologic Study. Arch. Neurol. & Psychiat. 70:741–777 (Dec.) 1953.

202. Nonne, M.: Weitere Erfahrungen zum Kapitel der Diagnose von komprimirenden Rückenmarkstumoren. Deutsche Ztschr. f. Nervenh. 47–48:436–503, 1913.

203. Nuyts, A., Hoffman, G. R., and de Haene, A.: Lipomes intraduraux de la moelle cervico-dorsale. Acta neurol. et psychiat. belg. 60:955–962, 1960.

204. Odom, G. L., Woodhall, B., and Margolis, G.: Spontaneous Hematomyelia and Angiomas of the Spinal Cord. J. Neurosurg. 14:192–202 (Mar.) 1957.

205. Oljenick, I.: Intramedullaire gezwellen (diagnostiek en heelkundige behandeling). Nederl. tijdschr. v. geneesk. 80:1335–1342 (Mar.) 1936.

206. Opalski, A.: Studien zur allgemeine Histopathologie der Ventrikelwände. Ztschr. f. d. ges. Neurol. u. Psychiat. 150:42–74, 1934.

207. Padberg, F., and Davis, L.: Tumors of the Spinal Cord. I. Intramedullary Tumors. Quart. Bull., Northwestern Univ. M. School. 26:204–211, 1952.

208. Paillas, J. E., Dongier, M., and Badier, M.: Les tumeurs épendymaires géantes de la queue de cheval. Semaine hôp. Paris. 28:2899–2901 (Sept.) 1952.

209. Parkinson, D., Medovy, H., and Mitchell, J. R.: Spinal Cord Tumor in a Newborn. J. Neurosurg. 11:629–632 (Nov.) 1954.

210. Pasteels, J.: Les effets de la centrifugation sur la blastula et la jeune gastrula des amphibiens. I. Mécanisme de la formation des organes secondaires aux dépens de l'ectoblaste. II. Étude comparative de la sensibilité en fonction des stades et des espèces. III. Interactions entre ébauches primaires et secondaires. IV. Discussion générale et conclusions. J. Embryol. & Exper. Morphol. 1:5–24 (Mar.) 1953; 1:125–145 (June) 1953; 2:125–148 (June) 1954.

211. Pasztor, E., Paraicz, E., and Szénásy, J.: Über Rückenmarksgeschwülste im Kindesalter. Deutsche Ztschr. f. Nervenh. 182:45–59 (Feb.) 1961.

212. Peers, J. H.: The Occurrence of Tumors of the Central Nervous System in Routine Autopsies. Am. J. Path. 12:911–992 (Nov.) 1936.

213. Penfield, W.: The Classification of Gliomas and Neuroglia Cell Types. Arch. Neurol. & Psychiat. 26:745–753 (Oct.) 1931.

214. Penfield, W.: Cytology and Cellular Pathology of the Nervous System. Ed. 2, New York, Paul B. Hoeber, Inc., 1932, pp. 423–901.

215. Pette, H., and Környey, St.: Zur Kenntnis der Rückenmarksgliome mit Ausgang in Syringomyelie: Zugleich ein Beitrag zur diffusen meningealen Ausbreitung des Glioms. Deutsche Ztschr. f. Nervenh. 117/119:371–408, 1931.

216. Peyton, W. T., and Baker, A. B.: Epidermoid, Dermoid and Teratomatous Tumors of the Central Nervous System. Arch. Neurol. & Psychiat. 47:890–917 (June) 1942.

217. Poser, C. M.: The Relationship Between Syringomyelia and Neoplasm. Springfield, Ill., Charles C Thomas, Publisher, 1956.

218. Pugliese, V.: Quoted by Sperling, S. J., and Alpers, B. J.[268]

219. Queckenstedt, H.: Zur Diagnose der Rückenmarkskompression. Deutsche Ztschr. f. Nervenh. 55:325–333 (Dec.) 1916.

220. Quincke, H.: Ueber Hydrocephalus. Verhandl. d. Kong. f. inn. Med. 10:321–339 (Apr.) 1891.

221. Ramamurthi, B., Anguli, V. C., and Iyer, C. G. S.: A Case of Intramedullary Neurinoma. J. Neurol., Neurosurg. & Psychiat. 21:92–94 (May) 1958.

222. Rand, R. W., and Rand, C. W.: Intraspinal Tumors of Childhood. Springfield, Ill., Charles C Thomas, Publisher, 1960.

223. Ranson, S. W., and Clark, S. L.: The Anatomy of the Nervous System. Ed. 10, Philadelphia and London, W. B. Saunders Co., 1959.

224. Rasmussen, T. B., Kernohan, J. W., and Adson, A. W.: Pathologic Classification, With Surgical Consideration of Intraspinal Tumors. Ann. Surg. 111:513–530 (Apr.) 1940.

225. del Regato, J. A. (Editor): Intracranial Tumors. Cancer Seminar, Colorado Springs, Colorado. 2:37–84 (Aug.) 1957.

226. Rhaney, K., and Barclay, G. P. T.: Enterogenous Cysts and Congenital Diverticula of the Alimentary Canal With Abnormalities of the Vertebral Column and Spinal Cord. J. Path. & Bact. 77:457–471 (Apr.) 1959.

227. Ribbert, H.: Über das Spongioblastom und das Gliom. Virchows Arch. path. Anat. 225:195–213 (Aug.) 1918.

228. Ricard, A., Thiers, F., and Bovet, M.: Résultats de 219 interventions pour tumeurs intrarachidiennes. Lyon chir. 48:527–534 (July) 1953.

229. Richardson, F. L.: A Report of 16 Tumors of the Spinal Cord in Children: The Importance of Spinal Rigidity as an Early Sign of Disease. J. Pediat. 57:42–54 (July) 1960.

230. Riggs, H. E., and Clary, W. U.: A Case of Intramedullary Sheath Cell Tumor of the Spinal Cord: Consideration of Vascular Nerves as a Source of Origin. J. Neuropath. & Exper. Neurol. 16:332–336 (July) 1957.

231. Ringertz, N.: "Grading" of Gliomas. Acta path. et microbiol. scandinav. 27:51–64, 1950.

232. Ringertz, N., and Nordenstam, H.: Cerebellar Astrocytoma. J. Neuropath. & Exper. Neurol. 10:343–367 (Oct.) 1951.

233. Ringertz, N., and Reymond, A.: Ependymomas and Choroid Plexus Papillomas. J. Neuropath. & Exper. Neurol. 8:355–380 (Oct.) 1949.

234. Riskaer, N.: Cysts and Tumors of the Septum Pellucidum. Acta psychiat. et neurol. 19:331–346, 1944.

235. Robineau, M.: Diagnostic et traitement des tumeurs de la moelle. Cong. Soc. internat. de chir. 2:575–622 (Mar.) 1932.

236. Rogers, L.: Tumours Involving the Spinal Cord and Its Nerve Roots: Bradshaw Lecture. Ann. Roy. Coll. Surgeons England 16:1–29 (Jan.) 1955.

237. Rohr, H., and Hoffman, W.: Rückenmarkstumoren mit Stauungspapille. Nervenarzt. 30:391–396 (Sept.) 1959.

238. Rokitansky, C.: Lehrbuch der Pathologischen Anatomie. Wien, Wilhelm Braumuller, 1856, 512 pp.; 1861, 557 pp.

239. Rosenthal, W.: Ueber eine eigenthümliche, mit Syringomyelie complicierte Geschwulst des Rückenmarks. Beitr. path. Anat. 23:111–143, 1898.

240. Ross, A. T., and Bailey, O. T.: Tumors Arising Within the Spinal Canal in Children. Neurology. 3:922–930 (Dec.) 1953.

241. Roussy, G., Lhermitte, J., and Cornil, L.: Essai de classification des tumeurs cérébrales. Ann. anat. path. 1:333–382 (May) 1924.

242. Rothmann, M.: Gegenwart und Zukunft der Rückenmarkschirurgie. Berl. klin. Wchnschr. 50:528–531 (Mar.); 598–603 (Mar.) 1913.

243. Russell, D. S.: Capillary Haemangioma of Spinal Cord Associated With Syringomyelia. J. Path. & Bact. 35:103–112, 1932.

244. Russell, D. S.: Polar Spongioblastomas: Their Place in the Glioma Series. (Abstr.) Proceedings Second Int. Congress of Neuropathology. Excerpta Medica Foundation, Amsterdam, The Netherlands, Vol. 1, pp. 259–260, 1955.

245. Russell, D. S., and Cairns, H.: Polar Spongioblastomas. Arch. histol. norm.y pat. 3:423–441 (Sept.) 1947.

246. Russell, D. S., and Rubinstein, L. J.: The Pathology of Tumours of the Nervous System With a Chapter on Tissue Culture in Relation to Tumours of the Nervous System [by] C. E. Lumsden. Baltimore, Md., The Williams & Wilkins Co. 1959.

247. Russell, J. R., and Bucy, P. C.: Oligodendroglioma of the Spinal Cord. J. Neurosurg. 6:433–437 (Sept.) 1949.

248. Saunders, R. L. deC. H.: Combined Anterior and Posterior Spina Bifida in a Living Neonatal Human Female. Anat. Rec. 87:255–278 (Nov.) 1943.

249. Sayre, G. P.: The Concept of Grading Gliomas of the Central Nervous System. J. Internat. Coll. Surgeons. 26:440–447 (Oct.) 1956.

250. Sayre, G. P.: Personal communication to the authors.

251. Scheinker, I. M.: Subependymoma: A Newly Recognized Tumor of Subependymal Derivation. J. Neurosurg. 2:232–240 (May) 1945.

252. Scherer, E.: Über die pialen Lipome des Gehirns: Beitrag eines Falles von ausgedehnter meningealer Lipomatose einer Grozhirnhemisphäre bei Mikrogyrie. Ztschr. f. d. ges. Neurol. u. Psychiat. 154:45–61, 1935–36.

253. Scherer, E.: Die Extramedullären pialen Lipome an der hinteren Wurzellinie des Rückenmarks (Kasuistischer Beitrag). Ztschr. f. d. ges. Neurol. u. Psychiat. 154:507–520, 1935–1936.

254. Scherer, H. J.: The Forms of Growth in Gliomas and Their Practical Significance. Brain. 63:1–35 (Mar.) 1940.

255. Scherer, H. J.: Critical Review: The Pathology of Cerebral Gliomas. J. Neurol. & Psychiat. 3:147–177 (Apr.) 1940.

256. Schirger, A., Uihlein, A., Parker, H. L., and Kernohan, J. W.: Hemangiopericytoma Recurring After 26 Years: Report of Case. Proc. Staff Meet., Mayo Clin. 33:347–352 (June) 1958.

257. Schlesinger, H.: Beiträge zur Klinik der Rückenmarks und Wirbeltumoren. Im Auftrage des Professoren-Collegiums der Wiener medicinischer Facultät aus anlass der Verleihung des "Oppolzer-Stipendiums." Jena, G. Fischer, 1898.

258. Schlesinger, H.: Die Syringomyelie: Eine Monographie. Leipzig & Wien, F. Deuticke, 1902.

259. Schultze, F.: Beiträge zur Pathologie und pathologischen Anatomie des centralen Nervensystems. Virchows Arch. path. Anat. 87:510–540 (Mar.) 1882.

260. Schultze, F.: Weiterer Beiträge zur Lehre von der Zentralen Gliose des Rückenmarks mit Syringomyelie. Virchows Arch. path. Anat. 102:435–451 (Dec.) 1885.

261. Scott, M., and Bentz, R.: Intramedullary Neurilemmoma (Neurinoma) of the Thoracic Cord: A Case Report. J. Neuropath. Exper. Neurol. 21:194–200 (Apr.) 1962.

262. Seifarth, G.: Das Neuroepitheliom des Rückenmarks im Lichte der organoiden Geschwulstbetrachtung. Virchows Arch. f. path. Anat. 316:149–186 (Oct.) 1948.

263. Shelden, C. H., and Bors, E.: Subarachnoid Alcohol Block in Paraplegia: Its Beneficial Effect on Mass Reflexes and Bladder Dysfunction. J. Neurosurg. 5:385–391 (July) 1948.

264. Shenkin, H. A., and Alpers, B. J.: Clinical and Pathologic Features of Gliomas of the Spinal Cord. Arch. Neurol. & Psychiat. 52:87–105 (Aug.) 1944.

265. Simon, T.: Beiträge zur Pathologie und Pathologischen Anatomie des Zentral-Nervensystem. Arch. f. Psychiat. 5:108–163, 1875.

266. Siwe, S.: Spinal Cord Tumors in Children. Acta paediat. 45:437–439 (July) 1956.

267. Slade, H. W., and Vinas, F. J.: Intramedullary Lipoma of the Spinal Cord. Neurology 6:449–452, 1956.

268. Sperling, S. J., and Alpers, B. J.: Lipoma and Osteolipoma of the Brain. J. Nerv. & Ment. Dis. 83:13–21 (Jan.) 1936.

269. Spurling, R. G., and Mayfield, F. H.: Neoplasms of the Spinal Cord: A Review of Forty-two Surgical Cases. J. A. M. A. 107:924–929 (Sept. 19) 1936.

270. Staemmler, M.: Hydromyelie, Syringomyelie und Gliose. Anatomische Untersuchungen über ihre Histogenese. Berlin, Springer Verlag. 1942.

271. Steinke, C. R.: Spinal Tumors: Statistics on a Series of 330 Collected Cases. J. Nerv. & Ment. Dis. 47:418–426 (June) 1918.

272. Stookey, B.: Intradural Spinal Lipoma: Report of a Case and Symptoms for Ten Years in a Child Aged Eleven; Review of the Literature. Arch. Neurol. & Psychiat. 18:16–42, (July) 1927.

273. Stookey, B.: Tumors of the Spinal Cord in Childhood. Am. J. Dis. Child. 36:1184–1203 (Dec.) 1928.

274. Storch, E.: Ueber die pathologisch-anatomischen Vorgänge am Stützgerüst des Zentralnervensystems. Virchows Arch. f. path. Anat. 157:127–171; 197–234 (Aug.) 1899.

275. Strauss, I., and Globus, J. H.: Spongioblastoma With Unusually Rapid Growth Following Decompression. Neurol. Bull. 1:273–281 (July) 1918.

276. Svien, H. J., Gates, E. M., and Kernohan, J. W.: Spinal Subarachnoid Implantation Associated With Ependymoma. Arch. Neurol. & Psychiat. 62:847–856 (Dec.) 1949.

277. Svien, H. J., Mabon, R. F., Kernohan, J. W., and Adson, A. W.: Astrocytomas. Proc. Staff Meet., Mayo Clin. 24:54–64 (Feb. 2) 1949.

278. Svien, H. J., Mabon, R. F., Kernohan, J. W., and Adson, A. W.: A Simplified Classification of the Gliomas, Based on the Concept of Anaplasia. S. Clin. North América, August, 1949, pp. 1169–1187.

279. Svien, H. J., Mabon, R. F., Kernohan, J. W., and Craig, W. McK.: Ependymoma of the Brain: Pathologic Aspects. Neurology. 3:1–15, 1953.

280. Svien, H. J., Thelen, E. P., and Keith, H. M.: Intraspinal Tumors in Children. J. A. M. A. **155**:959–961 (July 10) 1954.
281. Tamaki, K., and Lubin, A. J.: Pathogenesis of Syringomyelia: Case Illustrating the Process of Cavity Formation From Embryonic Cell Rests. Arch. Neurol. & Psychiat. **40**:748–761 (Oct.) 1938.
282. Tannenberg, J.: Über die Pathogenese der Syringomyelie, zugleich ein Beitrag zum Vorkommen von Capillarhämangiomen in Rückenmark. Ztschr. f. d. ges. Neurol. u. Psychiat. **92**:119–174, 1924.
283. Tarlov. I. M.: Ependymoma of the Filum Terminale. Arch. Neurol. & Psychiat. **32**:1045–1054 (Nov.) 1934.
284. Tauber, E. S., and Langworthy, O. R.: A Study of Syringomyelia and the Formation of Cavities in the Spinal Cord. J. Nerv. & Ment. Dis. **81**:245–264 (Mar.) 1935.
285. Teng, P., and Gordon, J.: Teratoma of the Conus Medullaris: Report of a Case. J. Neurosurg. **15**:569–571 (Sept.) 1958.
286. Tinsley, M., and McCoy, A. D.: An Intramedullary Epidermoid Tumor. Illinois M. J. **100**:200–202 (Sept.) 1951.
287. Turner, O. A., and Kernohan, J. W.: Vascular Malformations and Vascular Tumors Involving the Spinal Cord: A Pathologic Study of Forty-six Cases. Arch. Neurol. & Psychiat. **46**:444–463 (Sept.) 1941.
288. Urban, H.: Die Gewebsverschiedenheiten der Gliome und ihre klinischen Wechselbeziehungen. Frankfurt. Ztschr. f. Path. **46**:487–502, 1933–1934.
289. Verbiest, H.: Die Epidermoide des Rückenmarkes. Analyse eines Falles, zugleich Beitrag zur Frage der Entstehung der aseptischen Meningitis nach Epidermoidoperationen. Zentralbl. f. Neurochir. **4**:129–141 (July) 1939.
290. Verga, P.: Quoted by Sperling, S. J., and Alpers, B. J.[268]
291. Verhoeff, F. H.: Tumors of the Optic Nerve. In Penfield, W.: Cytology and Cellular Pathology of the Nervous System. vol. 3, 1932, pp. 1027–1039.
292. Virchow, R.: Die Krankhaften Geschwülste. Berlin, Verlag von August Hirschwald, vol. 2, 1864–65, 756 pp.
293. Von Remak, R.: Quoted by Bostroem, E.[23]
294. Vonderahe, A. R., and Niemer, W. T.: Intracranial Lipoma: A Report of Four Cases. J. Neuropath. & Exper. Neurol. **3**:344–354 (Oct.) 1944.
295. Vraa-Jense, G.: Angioma of the Spinal Cord. Acta psychiat. et neurol. scandinav. **24**:709–721, 1949.
296. Webb, J. H., Craig, W. M., and Kernohan, J. W.: Intraspinal Neoplasms in the Cervical Region. J. Neurosurg. **10**:360–366 (July) 1953.
297. Weber, E.: Die Teratome und Teratoide des Zentralnervensystems. Zentralbl. f. Neurochir. **4**:47–57 (Feb.) 1939.
298. Weicht, H.: Zur Morphogenese spinaler Höhlen-und Geschwulstbildungen auf dysraphischer Grundlage. Arch. Psychiat. **188**:99–119 (Oct.) 1952.
299. Weiss, L.: A Metastasizing Ependymoma of the Cauda Equina. Cancer. **8**:161–171 (Jan.–Feb.) 1955.
300. Wertheimer, P., Allégre, G., and Garde, A.: Les tumeurs ependymaires de la moelle et du filum terminale. Rev. Neurol. **82**:153–162 (Mar.) 1950.
301. White, R. J., Wood, M. W., and Kernohan, J. W.: A Study of Fifty Intracranial Vascular Tumors Found Incidentally at Necropsy. J. Neuropath. & Exper. Neurol. **17**:392–398 (Apr.) 1958.
302. Willis, R. A.: Pathology of Tumours. London, Butterworth & Co., 1948.
303. Wilson, S. A. K.: Neurology. Baltimore, The Williams & Wilkins Company, 1940.
304. Wolf, A.: Tumors of the Spinal Cord, Nerve Roots, and Membranes. II. Pathology. In Elsberg, C. A.: Surgical Diseases of the Spinal Cord, Membranes and Nerve Roots: Symptoms, Diagnosis and Treatment. New York, Paul B. Hoeber, Inc., 1941, pp. 231–364.
305. Wolf, A., and Wilens, S. L.: Multiple Hemangioblastomas of the Spinal Cord With Syringomyelia. Am. J. Path. **10**:545–567, 1934.
306. Woltman, H. W., Kernohan, J. W., Adson, A. W., and Craig, W. McK.: Intramedullary Tumors of Spinal Cord and Gliomas of Intradural Portion of Filum Terminale: Fate of Patients Who Have These Tumors. Arch. Neurol. & Psychiat. **65**:378–395 (Mar.) 1951.

307. Wood, M. W., White, R. J., and Kernohan, J. W.: Cavernous Hemangiomatosis Involving the Brain, Spinal Cord, Heart, Skin and Kidney: Report of Case. Proc. Staff Meet., Mayo Clin. **32**:249–254 (May 15) 1957.

308. Woodard, J. S., and Freeman, L. W.: Ischemia of the Spinal Cord: An Experimental Study. J. Neurosurg. **13**:63–72 (Jan.) 1956.

309. Woods, W. W., and Pimenta, A. M.: Intramedullary Lesions of the Spinal Cord: Study of Sixty-eight Consecutive Cases. Arch. Neurol. & Psychiat. **52**:383–399 (Nov.) 1944.

310. Wyburn-Mason, R.: The Vascular Abnormalities and Tumours of the Spinal Cord and Its Membranes. St. Louis, The C. V. Mosby Company, 1944.

311. Wycis, H. T.: Lipoma of the Spinal Cord Associated With Klippel-Feil Syndrome. J. Neurosurg. **10**:675–678 (Nov.) 1953.

312. Zimmerman, H. M.: The Nature of Gliomas as Revealed by Animal Experimentation. Am. J. Path. **31**:1–29 (Jan.–Feb.) 1955.

313. Zülch, K. J.: Über die geschichtliche Entwicklung und den heutigen Stand der Klassifikation der Hirngeschwülste (unter besonderer Berücksichtigung der Gliome). Zentralbl. f. Neurochir. **4**:251–272; 325–335, 1939.

314. Zülch, K. J. Über das "sog." Kleinhirnastrocytom. Virchows Arch. path. Anat. **307**: 222–252 (Dec.) 1940.

315. Zülch, K. J.: Die Hirngeschwülste. In Biologischer und morphologischer Darstellung. Leipzig, Johann Ambrosius Barth, Verlag, 1958.

INDEX